Pocket Practice Guides

Clients, Pets and Vets
Communication and management

Carl Gorman
BVSc MRCVS

Illustrated by Hayley Albrecht

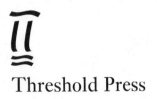

Threshold Press

First published in 2000 by
Threshold Press Ltd, 152 Craven Road, Newbury
Berks RG14 5NR
Phone and fax 01635-528375
email: publish@threshold-press.co.uk
www.threshold-press.co.uk

ISBN 1–903152–04–6

Designed and typeset by Jim Weaver Design
Printed in England by RedwoodBooks, Trowbridge

The Illustrator
Hayley Albrecht obtained an honours degree in silversmithing at
Loughborough in 1996 and has worked in this field and as an artist
ever since. She specialises in animal portraiture with clients in
America, South Africa, Ireland and the UK. She lives and works in
Berkshire in the faithful company of Boot and Tammy the dogs
and Sooty the world's most-adored pony.

Contents

(getting your money) – Worming – Flea treatment – Skin and ear cases – Neutering – Alternative therapy – Encouraging well-behaved pets

Introduction

My first morning in practice is still clearly imprinted on my mind. I'm not quite sure what I expected – a gentle introduction to the clients with another vet doing the talking, or perhaps a few clients with some instructions as to what to do with them. What I got was a consulting room, a busy practice with no one free to hold my hand and a waiting room full of clients unaware that they were my very first clients, all expecting me to deal with them competently and efficiently.

Calling the first client in, I desperately ran through the lists of possible ailments which might be presented. Gastric torsions, hepatic encephalopathies, cases of osteochondritis dissecans, persistent posterior pupillary membranes, atypical endocrinopathies, rabies. . . all jostled for space in my churning mind. The feeling of relief as the elderly gentleman placed his terrier on the table and asked me to clip its claws was terrific, but only temporary. My over-stretched memory was called into action again as I invited the next client in.

After surviving a surgery of vaccinations, sore ears, flea infestations and minor cases of diarrhoea, it dawned on me that each surgery might not in fact prove to be as nerve wracking as my final examinations. I also realised that in many ways I was in fact terribly unprepared for dealing with such mundane complaints. Veterinary school had turned out a practitioner fully primed to deal with a myriad of more or less unusual medical and surgical complaints. No one had really told me how to approach a simple case of gastroenteritis caused by the parts of the chicken vindaloo which no one else wanted, or how to advise an old lady of the best approach to worming her unhandleable cat. A full list of available drugs together with relative efficacies was readily available, but just how did one insert them into the cat?

A few months in practice brought home another fact of life. A vet's success with the public has little to do with how knowledgeable or skilful he or she is. Assuming a basic level of competence, a vet's reputation is far more likely to be based on client handling skills than on advanced veterinary ability. Combining both good bedside manner and a high medical success rate is a winning combination. It is, however, a vet's sensitive handling of euthanasia which produces the most letters of thanks, gifts and general pronouncements of satisfaction from the public. This, remember, is for a procedure with a one hundred percent mortality. I find this depressing in some ways, but it should bring home to us that dealing with clients and their pets in a gentle and sympathetic fashion is what will most enhance our reputation with the general public, even when we may feel we are failing medically.

Veterinary schools have to instil a vast amount of information into each successful veterinary student. Even our somewhat extended courses can seem too short a time to absorb everything. The actual business of dealing with common problems or communication with clients tends to be left for students to pick up when seeing practice. This has several disadvantages. Students tend to be far more interested in seeking out interesting or challenging cases rather than observing a vet's technique at the vaccination consultation. Everything is at once fascinating, confusing, exciting and sometimes boring. Without being told to watch out for consulting technique, methods of persuasion and other tricks of the trade, students often waste their first few sessions in a practice environment. Each student can only observe what is put in front of them. Practices and vets vary widely in their approach to the public and their relationship with them.

Clients in small animal practice are a varied bunch. They represent a complete cross-section of society. A successful vet must know how to handle the timid and the forthright, the knowledgeable and the foolish. Whatever else he or she may aspire to, a small-animal practitioner must be a performer, and each vet must put on tens of shows a day. A (successful) performance is necessary not only to improve your rapport with your clientele and to help your practice grow, but it will enable you to ensure that your patients receive the best health care and advice.

I wouldn't presume to tell each vet how they should treat their clients, but this book should provide points for thought and advice on what clients have been found to respond to. This will allow you to develop your own style, whilst saving you from having to experiment through years of experience before finding success.

1

Why do we need clients?

Why do we need clients?

Clients are a fact of veterinary life. They are at least as important as the animals we treat, and probably more so. Not only do they pay your wages, and those of your staff, but they will determine whether you are happy and fulfilled in practice. Deal with your clients well and you can look forward to each day's consulting. You will have the privilege of spending the day in the company of friends. Remember that in private practice it is clients and not you who decide the level of treatment their animals will receive – your professional life will be more satisfying if clients who like and trust you allow you to perform better veterinary medicine and surgery on their pets. Your staff will also enjoy their work far more if there isn't a 'them and us' attitude in the practice.

Do you remember a time, maybe when you were quite young, when the first spark of that burning ambition to become a vet flared up? Perhaps it was because you were terribly fond of animals that you set off down the long, and let's face it, difficult road. Maybe one of your pets was ill and helped by the local vet. Possibly you saw veterinary science as the route to fame and fortune. Having developed the ambition you may well have nurtured it by keeping pets by the score, by gaining work experience at kennels, veterinary practices, stables or zoos, and by taking a keen interest in natural history and how animals work. Having studied desperately hard and achieved top marks at A-level, you entered the hallowed portals of veterinary school. After a year or two you were probably even allowed contact with animals. As the years passed you gained clinical know-how and an expertise in handling animals and tending to their needs. Eventually you took and passed those final examinations and were released into the world of veterinary practice.

At what point during this process did you realise that treating animals was in fact going to be a virtual sideline to the much more demanding and time-consuming task of treating clients? Hopefully it was some time before you first walked into a consulting room on your own and dealt with the general public, but very often the realisation only dawns on a vet after a period in practice. Believe me, sometimes the most demanding orthopaedic procedure can seem like piece of cake when compared to the task of trying to explain to the venerable Mrs Bittenankles why a full program of flea control is necessary to eliminate parasites, and no, a bit of garlic won't work quite as well. (And that's when she *has* remembered to turn her hearing aid on.)

To work in practice, and particularly small animal practice, is to accept that every patient has at least one owner, and you are not going to get near the animal without dealing with the human first. It may seem to you after a short time in practice that your professional life might be much easier if you didn't have to deal with clients as well as their pets. Put this thought out of your mind. Such ideas can only lead to a poorer relationship with your clients. Once you start to resent clients, you have stepped on to a downward spiral leading to a loss of rapport with your owners and so to an unsatisfactory working life. Don't listen to dire warnings of a client's disagreeable manner or unpleasant attitude. Give each client you see a clean slate and more than likely you will bring out their better nature.

In short, clients are not a necessary evil of practice, but a necessary and enjoyable part of practice. Get used to them and appreciate them or you will condemn yourself to an unhappy career. After all, they do have their good points. Hardly any of them bite or scratch; they usually appreciate what you are doing for poor Pussykins, even if the cat doesn't; and if you treat them right they will often surprise you with a card and a box of chocolates or a bunch of flowers, just because you're doing your job.

The vet as social worker

By one of life's little quirks, the telephone number of our surgery is quite similar to the local social services number. As people rarely take in the first few words spoken when a phone call is answered, many of them

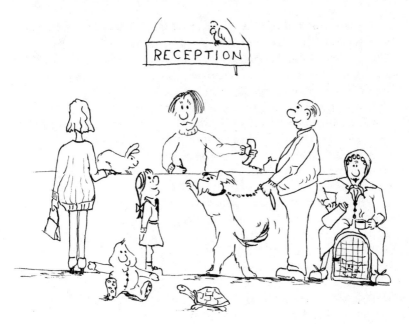

cheerfully ignore the fact that we are a veterinary surgery and proceed to tell us their woes. Often the requests are not really very inappropriate. Thus we may be asked to act as midwife as 'the baby's on its way', or we might be asked if we could 'send a nurse round to Auntie Flo – her leg's bad again'. Sometimes it can be quite hard to actually persuade callers that we are not really in a position to help. They probably think that we are just being evasive.

I often get the impression that many of those callers wouldn't be too disappointed if they did persuade our staff to turn out and minister to them. We are often being told that clients wished they received the same care, attention and affection that their pets are given. I do try to defend our hard-pressed medical colleagues, and I also point out that our clients do pay us to be nice to them, but nevertheless we should always treasure such praise and endeavour to live up to the good reputation that our profession enjoys.

My wife used to work in a practice on the south coast, where there is an even higher than normal proportion of elderly residents. A mature gentleman, Mr A, used to come in every week as regular as clockwork with his old terrier, Robbie. There was seldom a real problem with Robbie, week in, week out he would have his claws trimmed, his anal sacs expressed or pick up some wormers and flea treatment. One week the receptionist noticed Mr A sitting alone in the waiting room without his usual companion. 'Hello Mr A,' she called. 'Where's Robbie today?' 'Oh,' Mr A replied, 'Robbie's not very well today, so I left him at home.'

This tale and many similar ones come to mind almost daily as I see one or other of the regular clients we have who see the surgery as a place to talk, socialise or just get company. We provide a friendly face and a chat, and there are usually a selection of other animal lovers in the waiting room who can compare notes on their pets.

It is often said that dogs resemble their owners, and I'm sure you can all bring several examples to mind. The highly coiffured and perfumed Lhasa Apso (and owner); the grizzled old bandy-legged Jack Russell terrier (and owner); the well-dressed, long-legged, elegant standard poodle (and owner). Far more common, in my experience, is the dog which shares its owner's personality. This is entirely understandable since we are the pack leaders and role models for our dogs. They are highly receptive to our state of mind and take their lead from us. Thus a calm and outgoing owner will very probably have a well-balanced pet, while a highly strung and neurotic person will have a hard time trying to correct their dog's psychological problems. If you haven't already done so, you will certainly come across owners pleading with you to help them with Bodger's nervous nature and irrational fear of everything from fireworks to plastic bags. Frequently, you find yourself thinking that a prescription of Valium for the human half of the partnership would have far more beneficial effect than any treatment you give the dog.

It is important to appreciate the role that you have, and if possible to revel in it. Try not to think of these clients as time wasters or a nuisance, but as people who are just as entitled to your time and sympathy. Pets are a real boon, even a lifesaver to many lonely, depressed or troubled individuals, not only for the direct benefits of companionship that they give, but also because of the human contact that they encourage as well. Here is an opportunity with minimum demands on your veterinary skills to provide a tremendously valuable service to a portion of your clientele.

The vet's role and status in society

At the time of writing veterinary medicine is enjoying or enduring, depending on your point of view, an unprecedented amount of exposure in the media and literary worlds. Having started with the Herriot years, the enthusiasm shown by television for the veterinary profession in both fact and fiction has grown almost unbelievably, to the point where there have been evenings when it was hard to find a channel without vets appearing. Some satellite channels' programming seems to consist almost entirely of veterinary clinics from various corners of the world.

The popularity of the programmes reflects the British public's fascination with animals (don't flatter yourselves – the animals are the stars). As far as the pet owning public is concerned, anyone caring for a poorly pet is OK. Where for the average vet the fun of these programmes lies in snooping around other surgeries ('They don't keep patients in *there*, do they?') and criticising the treatment regimes of our media-exposed colleagues ('Well that one's bound to die, isn't it?'), the general public genuinely enjoys watching the succession of mundane tasks which we come to perform almost without noticing.

This level of familiarity with our profession brings mixed attitudes. This has always been the case. Not long ago the name of James Herriot would have formed a convenient expletive to be used by vets as they trawl in to the surgery at all hours of the night to see clients who assume that, just like James, all vets positively love being called out. What's more, the dirty subject of money was seldom brought up by the on-screen vet. Most clients probably also assumed that veterinary medicine still consisted of mixing various potions from dusty brown Winchester bottles; surgical instruments were sharpened on a strop each morning before being swilled briefly in a bucket of Savlon; and operations were carried out on the staff room coffee table by vets in mackintoshes and turned down wellington boots.

Nowadays clients have a certain degree of familiarity with our job. It used to be that on practice Open Days they were satisfied to see that we had cages to keep our patients, a couple of tables on which to put them and a plentiful supply of needles to go with those lovely bottles of drugs. Recently they barge in demanding to see the ultrasound machine and asking how many leads our E C G machine has.

In general the exposure has been beneficial. Clients are now aware that veterinary medicine is highly complex. They can see that the average veterinary clinic is much more akin to a hospital rather than the local G P's surgery. They are often encouraged to have more done to their pets because they have seen a similar case receiving 'the treatment' on television.

There has also been a demystifying of the profession, however. Seeing young vets making errors, admitting gaps in their knowledge and consulting with a budgie in one hand and a text book in the other makes all of us seem more human and less the infallible creatures of fiction. The profession, although still held in respect, is perhaps less likely to be held in awe. Personally, I don't think that this is a bad thing. I think that clients should feel comfortable with their vets and be able to discuss cases from a point of some knowledge. We in turn are more likely to have to justify our decisions, which I think will help us to make the right ones.

With the decline in farming and consequently farming practice there has been a great change in the public's perception of vets. Twenty or thirty years ago someone meeting a vet would expect to see a man in wellies with a green coat and a cap, and they would know that they had to be careful which hand they shook. (Not the green one.) Now we are seen much more as health care professionals for pets (i.e. child substitutes) and not only are women tolerated but positively welcomed. Deserved or not we enjoy a favourable status and a better level of affection amongst the population than our fellow professionals such as doctors, solicitors and dentists. Our clients regularly compare our clinics favourably with the local doctor's surgery ('I'd much rather come here than see my doctor if I were ill'). Our intellectual prowess can assume mythical proportions. I am often told that a vet's training is much harder than a doctor's because don't we have to spend 7/10/20/100 (delete as necessary) years in college. And we must be much cleverer than doctors because our patients can't talk and tell us what's wrong with them, although as I often point out, our patients are far less likely to swing the lead or try to con a sick note out of us.

The responsibility of the profession

You are fortunate to have joined a profession that is, at present held in such high esteem. We are seen as caring, dedicated, efficient and knowledgeable. We receive favourable reviews compared with our colleagues in the medical profession. I sometimes wonder whether patients would perceive that they got better service from the health service if they passed the doctor £15 or so at each consultation. Here perhaps is the essence of the matter – we provide a private health service for pets, and in a private sector a practice providing poorer service will be less successful than a more efficient, polite and caring one.

As a profession we shouldn't delude ourselves. Although we may bask in the glow of public admiration, ours is a service industry. Pets, however much loved, are a luxury item. Pet health care is even more of a luxury item. Furthermore, pets can't choose where they are going to go for their medical care. We must live up to our image for the good of the profession and take good care of our pet owners if we are to thrive.

The veterinary profession has to remain sensitive to the needs of clients, the whole cross-section of clients. Not just the well-to-do or well-insured who can afford for us to indulge in complicated medicine or surgery, but the pensioners and low-paid and those with families where a course of treatment for the cat after it's been in another fight may make a sizeable dent in the food or clothing budget. My family have a sizeable collection of cats, dogs, guinea pigs, fish, hamsters and sundry other pets. I try to stop and think as I lug home a bulging bag with vaccinations, wormers and flea treatments what the cost of this would be. If I weren't in the fortunate position that I am, would I really be able to afford to keep their preventative health care programme up, and what would I do if they were ill? The one area where veterinary surgeons tend to have a problem in public relations is financial. That vets' fees are high is a mantra repeated far and wide. We know that we provide good value for money, and that in order to give good veterinary care a practice must be well equipped, but the client is only interested in the bill he or she is paying at the time. The profession must be seen to give value for money. We must take care of our clients and nurture them. Never take them for granted.

While we are caring for our clients, we mustn't lose sight of our first responsibility, which is to the animals we care for. Alleviating their suffering must be our aim. In most cases this is an aim we share with our clientele, most of whom dote on their pets and would hate to see them uncomfortable or in pain. For reasons of ignorance, indifference or impecuniousness a fair proportion of clients will be unaware of, or pretend to be unaware of, conditions which do in fact cause quite marked discomfort. Those same clients who claim to have their pet's welfare at heart may well fail to recognise that limping isn't normal in old dogs or that a mouthful of calculus and gingivitis is very sore. The fact that pets rarely complain about chronic pain is used as an excuse to ignore it. When afflicted by a gradually worsening discomfort, animals are not aware that it could be made better. They simply assume that this is the way things are going to be, so what is the point of complaining. We must do the complaining for them, but in a sensitive way. No owner wants to be told that they are guilty of cruelty to their pet, and they won't thank you for telling them if you are too blunt. You must find the kindest path for pet and owner, but end up by helping the pet.

For the sake of the animals don't be too dogmatic. Not everyone can afford the most expensive treatment, regardless of how effective it is. We are aware that meloxicam or carprofen are potent, safe drugs for arthritis, but they also come at a premium. Phenylbutazone might be less effective and come with a list of side effects as long as a dachshund's spine, but it does have the advantage of costing pence per tablet. If a client genuinely can't afford the best treatment, be realistic. Would the pet choose to be in pain or risk the treatment? These are decisions you will have to make many times, with or without the help of owners.

Responsibility of the individual vet to the profession

As we have seen, by accident or design, the veterinary profession enjoys a favoured position, high in public opinion. True, this is in large measure due to the love of all things connected with animals which is prevalent in Britain. The generations of vets who have gone before you have also worked hard to earn the respect of society. Compassion, approachability, learning, efficiency, humour, value for money – all characteristics which the profession is known for and is proud of. We are known for thoroughness and honesty to the point where vetting has entered the language as byword for reliably checking. (Professional etiquette prevents me from pointing out what doctoring is a synonym for, let alone soliciting.)

On entering practice you are immediately reaping the benefits of the groundwork which has been done before you. You may see yourself on your first day at work as a bundle of nerves in a white coat, unable to imagine how you could say anything of value to any owner. Your clients, on the other hand, will see a knowledgeable young vet fully primed and prepared to deal with anything from a bleeding claw to a diabetic dog with Cushing's syndrome which has ruptured its cruciate ligament. You will be expected to give advice to breeders who have been producing puppies or kittens since before you were born, or to the owners of strange reptiles you had previously thought to see only on television or in a zoo. Amazingly enough, with very few exceptions, these people will listen to you and will follow any advice you might feel able to give them. This isn't because they trust you as such, but because they trust a veterinary surgeon.

In return for this great inheritance that you have been granted, you have certain responsibilities and duties. Your actions, words, dress, conduct and manner will all reflect not just on you, but also on the profession. To a certain degree you must strive to live up to the perceived public image of the vet. This is not to say that there is no room for individuality. Of course there is, and naturally it is good to make the most of your own characteristics and strong points. Just be aware of the accepted standards of conduct and behaviour. As a group so accustomed to positive press, we tend to react with panic and distaste to any publicity which shows us in a poor light. Stories of vets ripping off pet owners, carrying out illegal or cruel procedures or of insensitive disposal of carcasses – all reflect on each of us. Never underestimate the power of the media, incidentally. The briefest item on the news, or the shortest newspaper column buried in the middle pages will still bring a surprising number of comments and enquiries from clients. The internet is a new and insidious method of spreading rumour and adverse publicity. Many people seem to believe that because something is written down somewhere it must be true. The internet doesn't even benefit from the scant editorial control that some of our more lurid newspapers have. A well-produced web site is enough to give credibility to its content.

It doesn't take major misdemeanours or notoriety in the press to have an adverse effect on the reputation of the veterinary profession. If one is callous, unsympathetic, rude, inept or unreasonably expensive, another practice may benefit in the short term from an influx of clients, but we all drop a few notches in the opinion of a section of our clientele.

Stress avoidance

There is no doubt that veterinary medicine can be a very stressful career. Long hours, nights on call, the high expectations of clients and the trauma of cases that don't work out well – there are plenty of factors. Sadly vets are usually near the top of the table for suicides, although opportunity must play a part. Auto-euthanasia is easier for a veterinary surgeon or a doctor than for a hairdresser or an accountant. Alcoholism is also a fairly common affliction.

It is perhaps hard for those of us who don't suffer badly from stress and who don't experience deep depression or desperation to fully understand those who do. It is all very well to say 'If things are that bad, just stop doing the job', or 'Cheer up', but once despair sets in things seem to become more and more complicated.

The best advice that I can give is to practice stress avoidance from an early stage of your career. Much of the stress in our lives can come from the pressure of satisfying clients, coping with complaints or rudeness and worrying about cases. A good relationship with your clients will alleviate much of that stress. How much more pleasant is a scenario where everyone is on the same side, as opposed to a 'them and us' situation. You will still have occasional owners who are habitually unpleasant, rude or complaining, because they are a cross-section of society, and as is often said 'it takes all sorts'. Ask yourself this though: if Mr Nasty is sharp with you to the point where you take offence, and it preys on your mind, gnawing at you for hours or days afterwards, who is it who suffers? Not Mr Nasty, that's for sure. If you can forget it instantly, then no one is any the worse off. Try to shrug unimportant irritations off.

Don't ignore complaints or genuine grievances, or you will miss an opportunity to improve your practice. If they are unfounded, however, as they often will be if you are conscientious and follow good practice, then there is no reason to let them trouble you. If they are based on good grounds, then aim to only have a particular complaint once, as you will have corrected the factors which have lead to it.

It is important to have interests outside practice to allow your mind a complete break from your working life. Ideally activities where one mixes with non-veterinarians will facilitate this. Physical activity is particularly good at anaesthetising the mind. A fit body does also seem to help in coping with mental stresses and strains. When on holiday or away for a weekend, try not to think of practice at all. There is little if anything that one can do to affect the practice while away, and it will actually continue to run quite well without you. Worrying or fretting simply tires the mind, where a break should enable one to return completely rested and eager for action.

Above all, don't keep things to yourself. Problems and worries which seem almost insurmountable when viewed in isolation often melt away when shared and discussed. Colleagues can be very understanding and supportive. There is rarely a problem you will have that hasn't already been experienced and solved before. And keep a sense of humour. After all a trouble shared is a trouble doubled. That doesn't sound right; where's that calculator?

Benefits of good client relations

The social benefits of getting on well with clients are clear. Stress avoidance, as we have said. Being able to spend your days amongst friends, which is important when your hours are long. The likelihood of social contact outside work. A reduced incidence of complaints and niggles.

The professional benefits are also great. Not just the thriving practice, increased client base and higher income you will enjoy, although that can't be bad. Good relations lead to a mutual trust, so that clients will be patient and understanding, while you can expect them to follow instructions and return when they are supposed to. Happy and trusting clients are going to allow you to carry out far more in the way of investigation, quality medicine and intricate surgery. In effect having good client relations is the route to a happy and fulfilled career, and will allow you to develop your professional skills to boot.

Pets need vets?

One of the professions mild attempts at self-publicity produced the slogan 'Pets Need Vets' which could be seen on the odd T-shirt or car sticker. Being somewhat realistic, it was obvious to me that this was only half of the story, and I lived in expectation that I would one day open the door to the waiting room to find a motley crew of cats, mongrels and canaries wearing little coats with 'Vets Need Pets' emblazoned across them.

So, let's be honest: vets need pets, but pets don't get a say in where they receive their medical care, and few of them carry much cash. So, even more than pets, vets need clients, and don't forget it.

- Pets are all very well, but clients choose vets and pay the wages
- Clients often need therapy more than their pets do
- Vets enjoy a favoured status in society which we must try to live up to
- Sir Isaac Newton said 'If I have seen further, it is by standing on the shoulders of giants'; never forget that you owe much to the vets who have preceded you
- Good relations with clients are the key to a happy career

2

Making clients feel at home

Having the right state of mind

Having established and come to terms with the fact that clients are going to be a necessary and major part of our working lives, we must try to make them feel welcome in our environment. It is a natural trait of animal behaviour, humans included, to feel more confident and secure in our home territory, and conversely rather nervous and defensive on someone else's patch. We will tend to feel comfortable in our practices through familiarity, and this may cloud our perception of the nature of the practice. What we may find a cosily tatty warren with plenty of bolt holes for staff to hide from those nasty clients, our customers may see as an untidy, inconvenient and unwelcoming surgery which instils little pride or loyalty in them. Don't underestimate the value of the pride factor. We all like to feel that something we are using is a little better than the average, whether it be our car, our hi-fi, our holidays or our veterinary practice. And if a client feels proud of the place to which they take their pets, they will want their friends and acquaintances to go there too. No publicity is more effective or trustworthy than word of mouth. That applies as much to losing clients as gaining them – your pet owners are just as susceptible to the words of praise that their friends are spouting about the practices they visit.

So first of all, be prepared to see the practice, and particularly the 'front end' where clients are usually to be found, from the public's point of view. Spend time imagining what it is like to be a worried owner with a sick pet coming through your doors. Is the atmosphere welcoming, reassuring, comfortable? Or is it harsh, impersonal and unfeeling? Clients are rarely aware of your and your colleagues' clinical expertise. In general they are unlikely to make much distinction in terms of the surgical skills required between a cat spay and a triple pelvic osteotomy. What matters to them is the way that they and their pets are handled.

Practice ambience

For many a trip to the veterinary clinic is a pleasant social occasion. While you are wrestling with the problems of your community's pet population, their owners will be enjoying a chat, catching up with old times, comparing pets with each other and generally making themselves comfortable. This is good. Keep this in mind. If they are happy they will be like putty in your hands, and may even forget to pass the ritual complaint about the cost of keeping Bonny's vaccinations up-to-date, or to bemoan the lack of a national health service for pets. To achieve this they need a comfortable environment.

By now you will all be aware that nothing is more important to the health of certain pets, such as reptiles, than the habitat and conditions they are provided with to live in. Give them a spacious home, not overcrowded, warm but not too hot, correct humidity, pleasant lighting which is bright but not overpowering, a few things to look at and play with and protect them from stress and the reward will be happy, healthy scaly creatures. This is probably the only

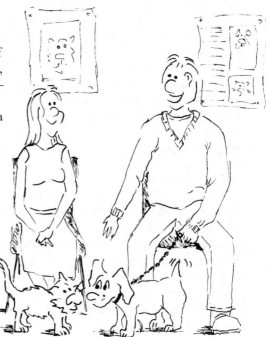

time that I am going to advise you to see your clients as cold-blooded reptiles, but you can see the similarity. The practice should be comfortable for both staff and clients.

Start outside of the building. I appreciate that there is probably little that you can do to remedy insufficient parking space. It is inevitable these days that the vast majority of clients in most practices will arrive by car. A sufficiency of parking is an important factor in people's assessment of a practice. You may not have the space to be able to produce ten extra spaces but it is possible to make the most of what you have. Marking parking spaces out improves the efficiency. Without marked lines many people seem to need to exercise quite a large exclusion zone around their vehicle. Whether this reflects on their confidence in their own ability to manoeuvre or everyone else's, isn't really that important. If staff cars are taking up several spaces, try to encourage members of the clinic to park outside the practice car park if feasible. It might be a minor irritation to have to walk a few yards more, but rather a staff member do it than an owner with a geriatric arthritic retriever or three cat baskets in tow. Altering the flow of clients to the practice can also be helpful. Schedule the dropping off and collecting of in-patients at different times to the consulting hours.

Make sure that the practice grounds and building are neat and presentable. Keep vegetation under control so that it doesn't present an irritation or even a danger to visitors. If there are areas prone to flooding or becoming muddy, consider what can be done to minimise the inconvenience that this causes. Keep signs clean and neat, and keep the décor presentable. Have sufficient lighting to ease use of the building on dark winter evenings or out of hours.

The entrance to the practice and the waiting room should also be kept well decorated and tidy. Too spartan an environment is probably less popular and comfortable than a mildly scruffy waiting room with posters overlapping on the walls. A note here – posters are not an alternative for wallpaper and paint. Try to keep posters topical and well rotated, so that it looks as though you have put them up for a purpose. Keep them well presented and tidy. The same goes for notice boards. If you rarely change posters and notices then they will become part of the wall as far as clients are concerned. They won't bother to read them and you will miss a valuable marketing and information tool.

Comfortable seating without crowding should be provided. If there is sufficient space, a separate area of the room for clients with nervous cats, birds or aggressive dogs (or children) is a good idea. Any areas for waiting room sales need to be well presented, attractively lit and regularly maintained. No one is going to be keen to buy tatty-looking merchandise or food covered in layers of dust.

Poor old doctors – the public image of the average G P's surgery is a rich source of items for our consideration and comparison. Often the doctor's reception desk looks rather like a Beirut bunker. Patients must feel they have to negotiate a minefield and strategically-placed barbed wire in order to approach a fox-hole of an office. Timidly they announce their arrival to hard-hatted receptionists who look ready to slam shut the sliding glass windows at the first sign of trouble or dissent.

We want to welcome people to our reception areas. A low wide desk which provides plenty of room for clients so that they don't have to queue in a line is ideal. The receptionist should be clearly visible at all times. Psychologically, a barrier between staff and clients can lead to a confrontational approach. Without the prop of a tall counter or a closing window, staff and clients tend to feel much more at one with each other. Sufficient staff to process clients rapidly and avoid log-jams at the desk are vital.

Hopefully by now you will have soothed, unstressed clients seated in comfort feeling good and ready to prove a most receptive audience for the main event. (That's you, by the way.)

Surgery pets

It is somewhat of a blow to one's confidence in a service provider if that individual doesn't have at least a token sympathy or familiarity with one's particular problems. Thus to take advice from a garden expert who lives in a flat feels rather strange. What do they know of soil conditions, compost heaps and galloping greenfly? How can they share your concerns about shady and sunny flowerbeds without having first-hand experience? How about buying meat from a butcher who is vegetarian? What sort of advice can he give you about the tastiest cuts, or the importance of marbling in your beef joint?

Similarly it always gives a client a little more confidence in their veterinary practice if they know that ownership of a pet or pets is involved, together with the intimate appreciation of the pleasures and anguish that this entails. For this reason I would strongly recommend that some pet animals are on view in the practice. These may be pets belonging to staff, bought for the clinic, or waifs and strays picked up along the way.

It never does any harm to let clients see these pets and follow their progress. They become quite attached to them, and it forms an extra bond between client and practice. Not all surgeries have the facilities to keep a practice cat, let alone a dog. Birds, fish and small furries do form a useful alternative, especially if the practice has an interest in exotics, when the animals provide free advertising and a big fillip to the confidence of owners.

Something a little out of the ordinary always provides an extra interest. One of my first surgery pets was a budgie called Paxo given to me by a client because both his feet were paralysed. To help him cope we padded his perches until he was able to balance on them and he proved a very cheerful member of staff. He was very useful as an illustration to owners of various aspects of bird keeping, including how to cope with disability. He had another important role to play in the practice: his cage was often kept in the prep room, and he provided a perfect distraction for cats as they were anaesthetised. We seldom had to struggle with one. Paxo would always strike up a furious racket whenever we answered the phone, and many a client would ask after him when they heard his chattering.

Other pets to grace my practices have been finches, parrots, rats and fish. Our present fish are large and full of character, entertaining both clients and their pets, as well as demonstrating that we are capable of keeping and growing exotic fish, and so able to dispense useful advice.

Staff selection and training

Staff that are going to come into contact with the public, and in most practices that means all the staff, must be able to present a consistently friendly and welcoming front. A member of staff who is excellent at other aspects of their job will not do the practice any good if they cannot interact well with clients. A client can't tell from meeting or speaking with a nurse that she is tremendously dedicated, very bright and able to work miracles with her patients. All they will see is how she deals with them, and possibly their pet, at the 'front end' of the clinic, or on the telephone. It is not enough to avoid being rude or impolite, a client has to be made to feel comfortable and important.

Some people are incapable of dealing with the public. They may have an unpleasant character, or more frequently simply feel uncomfortable talking to people. They may be shy or have poor interpersonal skills. Sometimes they feel very happy with animals, but are poor at coping with humans, hence they would like 'to work with animals', and may even be very good at the work. They are unlikely to be a great asset to the practice, unless the practice is large enough to accommodate them in roles which involve no contact with the public. Training and encouragement can help to improve the situation, but it is far easier to acknowledge from the outset that public relations are vital and avoid employing such staff.

At the least employees should be happy to deal with clients, capable of politeness, compassion and humour however stressed they are. Ideally they will thrive on the contact, enjoying the company of clients and welcoming them as if they were guests round for a social visit rather than carrying out a commercial transaction. This is obviously more important for reception staff than the back-room workers, but nurses should be encouraged to interact with your clients. A popular staff will be invaluable to your practice.

The practice's attitude to clients

In the middle years of this century, radio presenters working for the BBC were expected to wear evening dress when at the microphone, despite the self-evident fact that their listeners would never know what they were wearing. Common advice in training seminars on telephone manners is to always smile when speaking to clients.

Two examples of how getting the right attitude behind the scenes is important. What's more, it works. If you feel disinclined to try the evening dress wheeze, then have a go at smiling the next time you talk to a client, or even your mother-in-law, on the phone. And once you have discovered that it does help you to be more pleasant, adopt this as normal procedure. Smiling is a tremendous way of improving your state of mind, whether on the phone, in the middle of a fiendishly tricky piece of surgery or meeting clients.

Imagine this scenario: you have had a busy night on call, the telephone bill arrived before you left home, one of your colleagues is off sick so you'll be covering his duties as well. Before you see your first client, a new one to you, the receptionist says, 'Mr Beast wants to see you this morning. He's not happy with the way the treatment has been going.' Glancing at the card you see a selection of the practice's code acronyms or symbols which signify that the client is Satan in an anorak. You then open the consulting room door to call Mr Beast in. What chance does the poor client stand? You are primed to dislike him and to be on the defensive from the outset. He won't get the opportunity to develop a relationship with you, and will continue to be a disgruntled client.

In every clientele there will be popular customers and unpopular ones. It is natural for staff to feel defensive or outraged when clients are short with them or raise complaints or question the treatment their pets receive. It is vital to learn to cope with these feelings, not to let them influence dealings with the public and not to let them prejudice staff against certain owners. All staff, including the veterinary personnel, should be discouraged from discussing clients in a derogatory manner, or from making fun of them. It all may seem harmless enough at the time, but such behaviour cannot help but influence you and them when they come to deal with these individuals. Avoid the siege mentality, the 'them and us' syndrome. Try to look upon your clients as your friends, as valuable allies in the practice's quest to look after it's animal patients.

Just as talking in an adverse way about a client will, probably unfairly, prejudice you against them, the use of codes on cards to 'warn' vets about certain clients should be discouraged. Even if someone fails to strike up a good relationship with one vet, it doesn't follow that they will automatically clash with the next one they see. Give every new client you meet a chance. Don't prejudge. And even if you find that they are not your cup of tea, there is never any harm in being pleasant, understanding and polite. Clients may be unpleasant or abrasive for many reasons. You should be prepared to understand this. They are in any case in a stressful situation – their pet is unwell, they are out of their home environment and they are going to have to part with money. They may have had a bad day. Their house may have dry rot. Someone might have just scratched the side of their new Mercedes. They may have suffered a bereavement. They may not have benefited from a bereavement. It matters not – what is important is that you are generous enough of spirit to appreciate that there are many reasons for being cantankerous, and there is no need to respond in kind. Even if a client is a genuine bad apple, keep on smiling. Believe me, it may take years, but persistent pleasantness will break down the hardest of hearts. There is a certain satisfaction to be had when you get the first smile or thanks from a particularly hard case.

Remember too that clients have a perfect right to complain. A practice should never be so blinkered as to ignore this fact. Complaints may be justified or spurious. Often they simply arise from misunderstandings. Learn to listen to them, consider them and address them. It may simply involve explaining a course of action to a worried client, or it may involve putting an error right. Always be prepared to accept that errors can be made. Even if you don't always admit this to the client, don't try to fool yourself. Dealing well with complaints will usually not only satisfy a client but bind them more firmly to your practice.

Take some time to sit in the waiting room and observe the way that the clinic handles clients. Encourage other staff to do the same thing. Get everyone to try and imagine how they would be dealt with if they were a client. If you can all honestly say that you are not just satisfied with the client handling, but that you would get positive feelings as a member of the public using the practice, then many congratulations.

Dress code

In my early days as a practice owner, I spent many weekends at the surgery carrying out maintenance and DIY. There have been occasions when I have arranged to meet emergency cases at the clinic, and the owners have walked in to see me kitted out in blue overalls with paint liberally splashed over me, or even worse with sleeves rolled up and a drill in one hand and a hammer in the other. After trying to walk past me or perhaps asking me to locate a member of the practice, the realisation would dawn on them that they were expected to entrust their precious pet to this workman. I think that they did accept that I was a vet in the end, although the fact that I had to supplement my income by doing odd jobs obviously shook their confidence somewhat.

The point is that the public expect to see professional people dressed in an appropriate fashion. This conflicts a little with the modern trend to wear rather more casual clothes. The form of dress worn by vets when on continuing education courses has even been the cause of some extended correspondence in the veterinary media. As ever, the older and younger generations have tended to line up on opposite sides. The argument on one side goes that if one is dressed in an appropriate and tidy fashion one will be in the right frame of mind to concentrate and make the most of the sessions. The casual camp counters this with the contention that by being comfortable in body their minds are free to concentrate on assimilating knowledge. This debate extends to the daily clothing of vets in practice.

I don't wish to comment on the above debate, except to say that things can be taken too far. I once went for an interview to a practice where the partners consulted in pin-striped three-piece suits. To visit them must have felt much the same as to visit one's solicitor and see him wearing a green coat and a rectalling glove.

I am not going to suggest that wearing proper shoes and a tie will improve your clinical skills or ability to do your job, but then those are not really the subject of this book. Client relations, on the other hand, are. Most clients are going to feel at least a little reassured to see a veterinary surgeon dressed in the manner that they would expect, just as they like to see nurses in uniform. T-shirts, jeans, trainers and other more exotic clothing will, rightly or wrongly, diminish you in their eyes. Since it is necessary to have a client's confidence if you are going to be allowed to care for their pet, perhaps wearing the correct attire will help you to perform your job better after all. There is no need to be uncomfortably formal, but avoid looking casual, messy, slovenly, unhygienic or too experimental. Remember that you may be called upon to give bad news at any time, or to put someone's pet to sleep. As ever, think of things from the client's viewpoint and think of what you would like to see if you were in their shoes.

How familiar should you be?

Many clients visibly struggle when they try to find a suitable means of address for the vet. Often 'Doctor' will slip out almost involuntarily. We used to have a reasonable number of American clients who would routinely address us as 'Doctor'. This combined with the fact that they tended to find our bills ludicrously cheap and that they always wanted everything done for little Tiddles, tended to endear them to us somewhat. Our colleagues in the dental profession have recently decided to allow themselves the courtesy title of Dr. I like to think that we are secure enough of our worth not to need such a psychological crutch.

In our practice we tend to allow clients to choose whether to call us by our first names or to address us as Mr or Mrs (or Miss) Vet. When introducing ourselves in person or on the phone we will tend give our full names, and our Christian names are on our name badges. If one enjoys the confidence and respect of one's clients, I feel that it is unnecessary to insist on them using a formal approach when talking to us. Many individuals will however feel more comfortable referring to you as Mr, Miss or Mrs, however, which is fine. Our intention is to get to know our clients well and to try to make them feel like partners in the practice, rather than simply paying customers.

When addressing clients, we refer to them as Mr or Mrs Whatever, until they indicate that they would like us to use their first names, which many of them do. You can't be expected to remember everybody's Christian name, so a surreptitious note on the card or computer screen is invaluable.

The aim is to produce an atmosphere at the clinic which is comfortable for clients. They should feel that they have a good relationship with their vet, and feel that the vets can speak to them on level terms, not from some lofty pedestal.

The advantages of friendly relations with clients

Establishing a camaraderie with clients brings many benefits. In your personal life, you will be a member of your local community, and a well known one at that. You will see clients in most of your areas of social recreation. A friendly approach to clients within the practice will reap dividends outside it. Through your work you will know members of most sports and social clubs in the area, there will rarely be a pub you visit which doesn't contain a client or two, and the same is true for whatever social pursuits you favour. If you are seen as pleasant and approachable, your social life will be so much the easier.

In the workplace, establishing warm relations with clients leads to an invaluable mutual trust. Your clients will see their relationship with you as important, and will lend extra weight to the advice you dispense. They will be more inclined to allow you to perform a range of services for their pets, whether they be investigations, surgical procedures or lengthy courses of treatment. They are also going to be more patient with you when a case proves to be drawn out

Complaints will be much less likely. This is partly because of a reluctance to question a 'friend', but also because most complaints arise from poor communication, something you and your client have hopefully been able to overcome. Your friend the client is much less likely to seek a second opinion. At least they will probably let you know that they would like one, rather than sneaking off to a neighbouring practice and allowing the veterinary surgeon there to break the news to you. The client will benefit as well. You may be able to refer them to a colleague in the practice who has an expertise or more experience in that particular field, saving them money and the practice a client. If they do need referral, then you will be able to send them to a genuine expert and have the benefit of writing a full history of the case, in terms which shed the best light on your sterling efforts thus far. The pet then has a reasonable chance of further progress being made, rather than being shifted to a vet of similar expertise and skill to yourself who will quite possibly make little further progress with the case, yet feel justified in repeating many of your investigations and charging accordingly and get to keep a client who is often too embarrassed to return to their original practice, even if they'd like to. The trick with second opinions is to launch the client before they jump, but more of this later.

Should the worst come to the worst, and it will sooner or later, a client who addresses you by your first name and sees your relationship as warm and rewarding is far less likely to resort to such sanctions as legal action if they feel they have been wronged. You will at least have the chance to put your side, and to do what you can to placate the client.

Inevitably, although I hope that you will attain affectionate relations with a large proportion of your clients, there is some insincerity in this friendly approach. If you have a large clientele, you will not be able to remember all your 'friends' in intricate detail. It is somewhat embarrassing for both parties when a jovial gentleman trawls into the waiting room, catches you at the reception desk and launches into an intimate conversation, only for it to be obvious from your desperate puzzled look that you really don't have a clue who he is. This situation can be made more excruciating, should you so desire, if you have put the gentleman's cat to sleep the day before, been given an expensive bottle of wine by him as a present or he turns out to be the senior partner's husband. These things will happen, so try to be ahead of the game. Unless very sure of your ground, don't talk to anyone on the phone or in person until the receptionist has placed their record card in your hand or you have looked up their details on the computer. You may now commence your communication secure that you know who you are talking to, which animal you are likely to talk about and which problem you will probably discuss.

The pitfalls of familiarity

Along with the undoubted benefits of close friendship with each and every one of your clients come some rather less popular accompaniments. I will list some of these and I am sure that many more will come to light as you continue your career. Do try to retain a sense of humour if you have any of these drawbacks inflicted on you. Don't lose your temper or complain. Clients, even the really, really annoying ones, don't set out to irritate you. Oh, I'm sure they will, but don't flatter yourself that you have been singled out for their attention. It's just their little way. There was a particularly awkward client who made our lives a misery by taking up hours of consultation time, being rude to staff (sometimes in the most personal way), insisting on talking to us at the most awkward times and trying to direct our treatment of her pets. On top of this, she compounded the crime by running up a huge bill which she neglected to pay for so long that we had to refer her to our debt collection agency. I know that we shouldn't have allowed her to build up the debt, but whichever vet was unlucky enough to have dealt with her on a particular day would probably have paid good money just to see the back of her. Eventually she had to obtain the services of a solicitor to sort out her financial situation, and we had to contact the solicitor to clarify our part in the proceedings. When we spoke to him and explained that we were the veterinary practice calling in relation to Mrs $!!*&*, he replied 'Oh, thank God! Are you going to put her to sleep?'

First and foremost is the question of finances. However familiar we are with our clients, they are paying customers. We need to ensure that we give them good service. It is not acceptable to think that as it's only Mrs Nice, she won't mind her appointment being late, or appreciate a follow-up call after an operation or any of a hundred details we would usually attend to. Equally, as we are giving top service, we should charge normally. This should apply even to friends and acquaintances outside of the workplace. Once you start down the path of giving discounts to one friend, where do you stop? Keep the financial side of your work rigid and consistent, and concentrate on providing a service which is value for money. You may find that clients who consider themselves to be on good terms with you will push for a little extra discount. In my experience most genuinely friendly clients don't try this one on. Explain that it isn't within your power to alter the pricing structure. If it is within your power to change pricing, tell them that the fees are calculated so as to be fair to all clients, leaving little or no room for manoeuvre.

Clients may try to use their good relationship with you to obtain favours from you – seeing them at awkward times, asking you to visit them 'on your way home', dropping off drugs, perhaps collecting or returning pets scheduled for surgery and various other little courtesies. You may or may not feel inclined to offer these extra services, depending on just how good your acquaintance with them is. If doing a favour isn't going to put you out too much, it can be a marvellous public relations exercise. The image of the caring vet calling round to the house in pursuance of his duties is a strongly positive one. Consider whether you are willing to set a precedent, willing to perform the task again in similar circumstances and whether it might lead to unreasonable demands on your time and good nature.

One sometimes irritating consequence of cultivating certain clients is that they may become dependent on you to the exclusion of other veterinary surgeons in your practice. They feel that because they like you, and you seem to reciprocate, that they would be much happier for you exclusively to deal with their pets. This, although at times flattering, is not normally a good thing. On the one hand it implies a lack of confidence in the other veterinary staff; on the other it can lead to problems when their pets need treatment and you are not available. Suddenly it can seem as though you should be feeling guilty for having half days, nights off and holidays. This isn't a completely simple problem to resolve. There are a number of benefits for both client and vet if a pet usually sees one clinician. A frequent complaint when second opinions are sought is that the client always saw a different vet at the previous practice, with the attendant difficulties in following the case, and an avoidance of responsibility, particularly if the case is not going smoothly. From a vet's perspective, following one's own cases through is easier and more satisfying, and should lead to a much more logical approach to each particular disorder.

There are various ways of ensuring that clients will trust the other members of the practice. Try to make it a rule that a particular disorder in a specific pet is seen by the same vet as far as possible. If the complaint is a new one, however, then another vet should be able to take it on. I am sure that vets are without exception courteous and complimentary when referring to other members of the profession, but it is worth emphasising that one should talk up the other vets in the practice. Don't stare at a card in disbelief, slap your forehead with an open palm and say 'WHY has she done that?', for instance. Enhance their reputations with praise, cover up any apparent mistakes (and remember that there is often a good explanation for even the most bizarre courses of action) and generally show every confidence in them. You may have individuals who specialise or have a particular interest in certain fields. If so, tell the clients that you will consult them for an opinion, or ask them in to examine the pet as well. Even if there are no specialists *per se*, consulting a colleague does your reputation no harm and shows that you all have faith in each other. Tell your clients when you are due to go on holiday if you are in the middle of a case, and suggest a colleague who can speak to them or continue treatment in the meantime. Do let your colleague know as well, so that they don't let you down by professing to know nothing at all about the case. Make copious notes about the treatment or investigations you were planning on the records.

You may find that you are called at home by some regular clients. This may happen because they think that you would like to speak to them, because they don't wish to talk to another vet, because they don't like what they have been told by another vet or because they just happen to have your number. Clients can obtain your number in various ways, ranging from the telephone directory to using the '1471' facility after you have called them on a previous occasion. Contacting vets at home is definitely to be discouraged, and you need not feel guilty about this. You do have to be tactful, however. Sometimes a simple explanation of the operating procedures of the practice are sufficient. Some clients assume that each vet is on duty all the time, and so it is quite legitimate to call you whenever they need to speak to one. Deal with their query if you can, then request that for their own and your convenience they call the practice emergency line in future.

If it sounds like they need to see a veterinary surgeon, offer to contact the duty vet and ask him to call them. This will only take a few minutes of your time, almost all clients are quite understanding and you have also managed to look concerned and efficient.

Another task that you may well be asked to perform for your regular pet patients is euthanasia. I do feel that if you have been seeing a pet on a regular basis and the owners like to see you, then you should make every effort to be available. Of course there will be times when a pet deteriorates rapidly and it is just not practical for you to be there, but in general the owners will derive some comfort at a difficult time if they know that the vet their pet is familiar with does the deed.

Meeting new clients

When seeing clients for the first time, take a moment or two to read their records and glean any information about them or their pets that you can. They will appreciate the fact that you are familiar with them and with Bonzo's little problem. Everyone likes to feel special, so spoil them a little. If they have been seeing another vet and she has passed information on to you, tell the clients. They like to know that the vets do actually communicate and that Bonzo has been deemed important enough for discussion.

If the clients are new to the practice, you must be even more welcoming and helpful. Give a good impression of yourself and the practice to bond them to you. Take the time to find out about them if you can, and what their pet owning history is. Have they others at home? Have they any special interests? Make them feel that this is the clinic and you are the vet that they have been looking for. Whether the client is new or not, don't leave them struggling to lift their pet on to the table. If you want the pet up, lift it yourself or offer to help.

Clients with new puppies or kittens offer an excellent opportunity to bond with clients. However hideous or attractive you find their little treasure, this is a creature that these people have found irresistible enough to bring into their lives. Gush over it with them. Act as though you are deeply envious of them – if only you had spotted the little darling first. . . . To many of us this behaviour comes naturally enough. After all, puppies and kittens are appealing. However, if you are not sincere, never mind. Just be convincing. You can then pass on all the practice doctrine on health care and the correct upbringing of mini cats and dogs. If they are too distracted to hear what you are saying, give them an information sheet with the crucial information.

Making time

We have chosen to work in a busy profession. There are many demands on our time – trying to keep up with consultations, finishing operating in time for a few minutes of lunch, catching up with test results, filling in insurance claim forms, making and fielding telephone calls – you get the picture. In each day we see dozens of clients and have to juggle several cases at once. As far as each client is concerned, however, they are the only case that you have to deal with. Their only concern is the well being of their pet; to make sure that it receives your full attention, and that it benefits from the best of health care. Your task, as part time magician and illusionist, is to make them feel that they are indeed your only concern, and all other cases take a subordinate place. To do this with one client is easy, but you must achieve this with each of your owners.

Although hard to do well, juggling clients effectively can be accomplished. When performed successfully, you will reap the rewards of having more loyal clients. Part of the act involves always appearing calm under pressure, which in itself sends out a very positive message to the client, who will see you as an unflustered and clear thinking clinician.

Firstly then, in dealings with clients, remember to smile. Harassed vets who are not keen to see or speak to clients can be expected to look flustered, frown and grunt a lot, and agreement to converse with a client is often proceeded by a tetchy sigh. Don't let your customers see this. They won't thank you for being made to feel a nuisance. They probably know that you are busy – they've seen *Animal ER* or whatever on the television. They want to know that you can cope. So, if a client is within earshot, smile at the receptionist or nurse who passes you the message that your presence is required. Even if the client in earshot isn't the one in question, act as though you would be delighted to speak to whoever is demanding your attention. Clients know that if you deal badly with another person, they are likely to receive similar treatment in their turn. Even if you are only asked to speak on the phone, smile.

Try to avoid using the practice's heavy workload as an excuse for forgetting to contact someone or to chase up a laboratory result. At best this simply says that the client is a low priority, and at worst they may decide to try a practice with a less hectic lifestyle. Ideally, don't forget to fulfil your obligations, even if it means using a few minutes of your time at the end of the day. If you have got behind with tasks, try to make it sound as if you have had the case uppermost in your mind. Perhaps it is taking a little longer than expected because of the complicated tests involved, or you are having to find a relevant article in a journal. If you really haven't got time to speak directly to the client, make use of your support staff, who have often got more time to donate to the client. It helps to reinforce the staff's importance in the practice, and they usually enjoy the client contact.

Even if you are in a tearing hurry, once you are with the client take a deep breath and appear relaxed. Don't give out signs that they are taking up too much of your time, or that you are not giving them your full attention. You will have to develop techniques to move them on in a reasonable time, otherwise all your other clients will be short-changed, but this can be done gently, tactfully and often without the client being aware that they are being gently hurried along. For the sake of your colleagues please develop methods of doing this, or you may pay for your popularity amongst clients with the frustration of your fellow vets.

Remember the personal touches. Call up with test results or to find how an animal is responding to treatment. Telephone owners to let them know when their pets have recovered from surgery, or how in-patients are progressing. I usually use a safety net by asking an owner to call at a certain time or date in case I am too busy or forget to call, but I then try to contact them before they contact me. Note on the patient's records that you have called, and the time of calling, should the owners be out. You can then immediately apologise to the client if they contact you first, and tell them when you telephoned them. Be sure that you don't do this in an accusing or self-righteous way; you are simply trying to let them know that they haven't been forgotten. If the client has an answering machine, use it.

To joke or not to joke

Sharing a joke with a client or pulling their leg is a good way of making them feel at ease and letting them know that they are more than just a passing customer. What is important is to pitch things at the right level. Depending on relations with each client, and their character, the right level

may range from deadpan serious to stand-up comic. I can think of clients
who quite like to be greeted with 'Not you again! If you bring Spot in any
more often I'll have to call the RSPCA.' Other clients might give a sniff
and turn on their heel.

Our antipodean locums often seem to get away with murder, dispensing
cheerful insults to pets and owners alike. In general clients see no harm in
an exuberant attitude to practice, but there are some clients and some occasions which call for a more sober approach, and it is up to you to gauge
your audience. Many a straight-laced elderly lady has been found to develop a twinkle in her eye when teased gently. Know when to stop and this
may prove one of your most useful weapons in the war to win clients over
to you.

Children

If anything is likely to send a chill feeling through the average practice staff
member it is the thought of one parent and an indeterminate number of
children invading the clinic. While the father concentrates on restraining
the dog or cat, the children are loosed upon the waiting room, other clients
and their pets and any surgery equipment that isn't locked up or electri-
fied. The brood distract their parents whenever questions are asked or
instructions are given. They ask staff questions, often, depending on their
age, in a language which appears to bear no relation at all to English. You
may find yourself staring in blank incomprehension at a two year old,
while its mother (who clearly thinks that you are being difficult) translates.
'Juliet said "Is Pickles going to die?", "Have you any sweeties?", "Haven't
you got hairy ears?" ' or some other disconcertingly direct statement. The
noise level in the practice seems to climb several thousand decibels and as
you leave the consulting room you may find that everyone else has discovered some important task involving earplugs and being far away, leaving
you to cope alone.

   If a parent complains to you that their dog seems to want to bite one of
the children, resist the temptation to tell it to join the queue. We may fondly believe that pets are more convenient, more loveable, better-trained
child substitutes, but in reality there is no substitute for children, at least
in their parent's eyes. If you want to keep your child-owning clients happy
you will have to adapt to their children. In doing so, you will make life
much easier for the practice.

   When making up displays of posters and on notice boards, cater for the
younger audience as well. Have some magazines and books available which
would interest kids. Pencils and colouring books, or printouts of the practice's

own design, usually go down well. If the clinic is fortunate enough to have room to spare, set up a corner of the waiting room as a kids' corner, with toys and activities. This may even remove the need for them to enter the consulting room – big bonus. Competitions and quiz sheets will occupy older children. Have a notice board where they can display pictures of their pets. A television and video tape recorder can be used to play animal-related video cassettes.

Find out if any of your staff have an affinity with children. Many are very good given the opportunity. For the sake of tranquillity it is worth letting them spend a little time entertaining young children or looking after infants while you deal with the parents.

Once the children have reached the consulting room (and with luck you will have enough entertainment outside to keep them in the waiting room) you are on your own. It isn't really practical to have toys and games in the consulting room, and any hold they had on the children's attention would soon be lost when confronted with the much more interesting array of drugs and equipment laid out before them. In order to do your job properly, you may need to be firm with the children. This is necessary not only for your sanity, but also from a safety aspect, so that parents should accept that Junior should stay on their side of the consulting room table. Once they are under control, don't ignore them. Young people are fascinated with animals and the veterinary profession, just as we were. Talk to them, explain what you are doing and answer their questions. Try to maintain a sense of humour when they tell you that Rolf Harris would treat a case differently.

If the children are manic, they will not only distract you, but also your client and patient. If necessary, take the pet to a quiet room with a nurse to examine it or to treat it. Consider either writing down your diagnosis and treatment plan or telephoning the owner later so that they can digest the information with a clear mind. You may want to suggest scheduling the next appointment for a time when the kids are at school or nursery.

Children are actually potentially very useful. For one thing they are all future owners of pets. Teaching them at an early age about health care will stand you or your successors in good stead in years to come. They are often very caring about their pets, and are likely to force their parents to take notice of problems, encouraging them to seek our advice. They are also good little spies. When mummy claims that the emaciated cat on the table has only been vomiting for a couple of days, little Treasure is likely to pipe up: 'No Mummy, Splodge has been sick for 3 weeks. And that medicine you got from Pets R Us didn't help. And you said we didn't need to get its vaccinations done this year. And you gave it that old tin of salmon you found under the stairs. And the other vets couldn't make her better.' Etc.

Get the kids on your side. They will spread the word at school so that their friends will want their parents to go to the 'nice vets'. They will ensure that your patients receive their medication at the correct time. To many children vets are the caring, patient, kind professionals that they read about and see in the media. You are like a doctor, but much more important because you are caring for their precious pet and if anything gets hurt it's not going to be the child. You benefit from a degree of hero worship before you have even started – don't let them down.

- A practice should be welcoming and provide a pleasant atmosphere
- Surgery pets present a positive perception of the practice
- Staff should be comfortable dealing with the public
- Avoid discussing clients in disparaging terms at any time – a positive attitude will give a positive image
- Dress like a professional – fulfil your clients' expectations
- A close, friendly relationship with clients brings many benefits
- Every client likes to feel like your only client

3

Making your message understood

Problems of misunderstanding

One of my favourite cartoons sits above my desk at work. In the first frame an elderly lady has brought her little old poodle to the veterinary surgery. It sits on the table and the vet is talking to her. 'Incontinence, failing eyesight, arthritis. . . I ask you Mrs Nibbles, is that any kind of a lifestyle?' In the second frame the elderly lady is laid out on the table with a syringe of pentobarbitone protruding from her, while the poodle looks on smugly from the floor.

Similar 'real life' stories abound. There is the one about the client who drops an ageing dog off at reception with the instructions that it has come to be put to sleep. The locum on duty duly complies, only to find the owner returning after lunch expecting to collect his pet. The dog usually has a sedative to have its claws clipped, which to the owner's way of thinking is being 'put to sleep', a slightly misleading euphemism which many veterinary staff take to mean euthanasia. Although the stuff of legend, I am sure that this and other similar stories are in fact based on actual occurrences.

Misunderstandings between clients and veterinary staff are at best embarrassing and inefficient, and at worst disastrous for the pet, the client and ultimately for you. Together with a lack of communication they are surely the most common reasons for second opinions being sought. Often the vet seeing the case as a second opinion will do no more than repeat the investigations and treatment that the first vet used, with in many cases no difference in outcome. In the second instance, however, the vet will probably tell the client exactly what he is doing, together with a reasonable expectation of the response to therapy and course of the illness. Result: a contented client.

In our working days we use a plethora of pharmaceutical and medical terms, acronyms, abbreviations, mnemonics and brand names. Although second nature to us, RTA, DOA, CCF, CRF, bid, eod, POM, PO, EUA, GA, luxation, enrofloxacin and propofol mean nothing to the average client. We have to make a conscious effort to ensure that we are understood, and that we don't use jargon to confuse and frustrate the people most concerned about their pets. Owners don't like to feel excluded from the treatment of their pets and the decisions that are made. Be sure that they have as much information as is appropriate to the client and the case, in a form that they can understand. I know that there exists a school of thought which basically considers that the less a client knows about what is going on, the less they can interfere and the less able they are to question a course of action, or to appreciate if things have gone wrong. This is unfair to the vast majority of clients, isn't appreciated and won't protect you should mistakes be made. In fact, the more that a client is involved in each step of the decision-making process, the more the responsibility for the case is shared. Thus even if things don't run smoothly, the pet's owner will have been aware of all possible pitfalls and should have accepted the risks. They are unable to do this if they are not fully informed of the state of play.

Missing the point

Don't make the mistake of assuming that just because you know what you mean when describing a disease or a course of action, that the client automatically does as well. They may appear to nod wisely and agree earnestly with you, but they will often misunderstand you completely. Clients commonly look horrified when you give them a syringe with which to dose their pet with oral medication. They are under the misapprehension that you want them to inject the animal with the drug – not something I'd like to see the result of if you've given them some kaolin. One of our clients was given some large bullet shaped tablets of kaolin and antibiotic to give his German shepherd which was suffering with a bout of diarrhoea. He returned a few days later and reported that the dog was much improved but that it would-n't allow him near its back end any more, so could he have a different medication. Intrigued, we questioned him further only to find that the gentleman had been under the impression that the tablets were pessaries and he had been gamely pushing them up a rather reluctant dog's bottom.

Another quite common situation occurs when you have discovered a ter-minal problem, particularly if the client has brought in the pet for a minor problem, or for its vaccination. The vet gently informs the owner of the fact that, for instance, the cat has a large tumour of the bowel palpable, it is inoperable, the cat is in discomfort, there are probably metastases and really it would be kindest not to keep the cat going. If the vet hasn't spelled out absolutely clearly that she means that the cat needs to be euthanased, and as soon as possible, she is quite likely to receive a reply along the fol-lowing lines: 'But he will be all right, won't he?', 'Shall we do his vaccination now then?', 'Does this mean I'll have to give him tablets?' or one of many questions which show that the vet has, in this case, failed to establish contact.

While on this tack, does this ring a bell? An elderly bitch with a rup-tured pyometra is brought in. She has peritonitis and is in shock, but she manages to stagger in gamely as many dogs do. She is rushed into the surgery for stabilisation and surgery. She receives the best attention and medication. Many hours are spent tending to her and repairing her. Eventually, three days later, she bounces out to the waiting room to be reunited with her owner, having come within a whisker of booking her room in the big dog kennel in the sky. The owner looks at her critically and her first comment is 'You haven't clipped her claws! That's what I brought her in for in the first place!'

How about the client whose dog has developed heart failure (or one of a score of other complaints). You stabilise the animal and give a course of treatment which enables the pet to behave in a normal fashion again, and you then don't see the owner or pet again for months, by which time the condition is as bad as ever, the month's supply of tablets which you pro-vided having long been used. 'Oh!' says the client, 'I thought you had made her better. I didn't realise that she had to take tablets for the rest of her life.' *For the rest of her life* is a phrase you are going to have trouble with. Most owners are quite happy coping with a five day course of drugs, but they do get worried when medication is going to become a permanent fea-ture of their relationship with their pet.

I, and you, could go on for pages detailing those little incidents which illustrate the different languages that vets and their clients speak. By all means chuckle over such stories, but remember that they don't demonstrate the clients' lack of intelligence or common sense, but our own failure to ensure that we have made ourselves clear and that there is no room for misunderstanding. At one level misunderstandings are amusing, but they are potentially damaging for pets and for you. They may lead to expensive procedures or tests being performed when the clients had no idea of their complexity or cost. They may lead to the wrong treatment, or even to euthanasia when it wasn't wanted.

Tailoring your language

Your clients represent the complete cross-section of society. It follows that they will have a widely varying level of intellectual capability. Consequently it is necessary for you to pitch your language and descriptive terminology at the level which each client will understand. I find that in general I speak one language to my colleagues and staff, and another entirely simpler version to my clients. Often it is actually harder to adequately describe what you want to in layman's terms, but blinding with science is pointless.

I will normally start simple and work upwards in terms of complexity if the owner has some medical knowledge or watches *Casualty* regularly. Never make assumptions about your client's level of competence, as you will usually be caught out. I once explained a patent ductus arteriosus to a most unprepossessing chap in simple terms which I thought that the average *Blue Peter* viewer would comprehend. After listening patiently to me, he gently informed me that actually he had been a consultant paediatrician at Great Ormond Street hospital, and had a little experience of such defects. Still, I would rather work that way round than take too much for granted. Sometimes doctors and vets who haven't worked in practice can show a very poor grasp of proceedings.

When at university, one of my friends was a French speaking Swiss student, called Charles. Another student reading modern languages and quite full of himself, was delighted to find a native to practice upon. After a few days of putting up with the language student spouting torrents of French in his direction at every opportunity, Charles had had enough. The next time he was assailed, Charles interrupted the student and in a clear unaccented voice pleaded: 'Speak English so that I can understand you!' Sometimes it is best to stick to simple, jargon-free language.

Don't be insultingly simplistic to your clients, but as you eagerly expound the various actions of ACE-inhibitors, or explain the complexities of enterohepatic circulation, just take a little time out to ensure that your audience is following you and understands the points you wish to

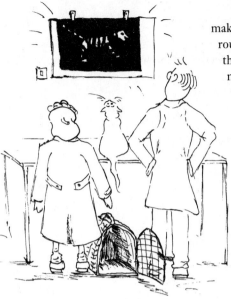

make. Avoid the somewhat easier route of not explaining anything to your client – the 'trust me' approach. I will admit that there are some sections of society who would appear not to have any interest in the whys and wherefores of diagnosis and treatment. They simply want you to get the pet better. Believe me, though, these clients are not very common. Trust them to have some interest in the case and get them involved.

Getting a meaningful history

As important as a physical examination, if not more so, is a good history. The art of history taking isn't always developed well at veterinary school. It is a skill which needs practice to perfect. When you are a student, you may either not get much opportunity to collect a history, or else you are left for half an hour to extract every last detail from the owner, from pet's date and place of birth and star sign, to its favourite colour and musical tastes. In a practice situation, you need a quick, relevant and useful history. This will very often tell you exactly what you are dealing with, enabling you to use the physical exam to confirm your tentative diagnosis. Do you remember those bacteriology practicals all those years ago? You would be presented with petri dishes containing four different bacteria, a brief history and a microscope. Your task was to identify the little blighters. If you were anything like me, the little spots and rods that were visible down the lenses all looked remarkably similar to each other. Fortunately, in most cases the little bit of history that was provided told you exactly what organisms you were likely to be staring at. Practice is just the same.

Now we come to the slight bug bear. Clients do, for some reason best known to themselves, often seem to do their best to mislead you or conceal information from you. It is almost as if they see the consultation as a little contest, whereby you have to use all your wits and skill to get a meaningful answer from them. Are these situations familiar?

Vet: 'What seems to be the problem?'
Client: 'I don't know. You're the vet; you tell me!'
(one of the few situations where I am perhaps slightly tempted to use Nembutal on a client)

Vet: 'How old is Poppet?'
Client: 'I don't know Doctor; we rescued her.'
V: 'Well how long have you had her?'
C: 'Seven years.'
V: 'And was she full grown when you got her?'
C: 'Oh no! She was only a tiny puppy.'

Vet: 'How old is Poppet?'
Client: 'Well we got her when our Julie got married and moved away.'

Client: 'He hasn't eaten anything for days.'
Vet: 'How often is he being sick?'
C: 'Five times a day.'
V: 'And what is he bringing up?'
C: 'His dog food, chicken, ham, his bones. . . .'

Another less than helpful situation is the husband and wife team. You just know as they walk in that they are going to contradict each other on every point, from what the pet eats, to how long it has been ill and what the response to treatment is. It never ceases to amaze me how one person can claim that the pet is now perfect, while the spouse will swear that the treatment has had no effect whatsoever. My advice in these cases is to make your own mind up, plucking the most likely facts from the dual stream of data.

At other times clients can display a spectacular lack of comprehension of the significance of certain symptoms shown. My wife had a very Pythonesque experience once. A gentleman brought in a box, which apparently had a cockatiel in it. 'I'm a bit worried about my bird,' he said, 'as I've heard that cockatiels can go into comas, and mine has been lying on the bottom of its cage.' 'How long has he been in a coma?' asked my wife. 'Three days,' replied the client, opening the box to reveal a decidedly deceased and somewhat stiff bird.

Be methodical and patient with clients. Try to keep them to the point. Develop your interrogation technique to ensure that you can extract the vital pieces of information that you need with or without the owner's help. Bear in mind that they won't always appreciate how important it is to know whether their pet coughs at exercise or at rest, or whether it has fits before or after feeding. They will often be upset or distressed, which can cloud the thinking of the best of us. Use an understanding approach to coax the information from them. The best history-taking occurs when the clients are mostly unaware that you are extracting valuable data from them. To them you are having a friendly chat, which relaxes them and helps to clarify the history. You, on the other hand, should be trying to find out what you want to know in the shortest time that is polite.

The advantages of getting your point across

If you are able to establish an effective two-way communication with your clients, this will bring several advantages.

You are doing a job, and should be earning money for the practice, so let's start with financial benefits. Well-informed clients will be a better investment for the practice. They will follow treatment regimes better because they know the reasons behind those regimes. They will opt for the better quality treatments when you consult them, because you have explained the benefits of such courses of action. They will be keener to have both initial investigations of illnesses carried out, and appreciate the need for repeating those investigations at regular intervals. They will be more inclined to follow your advice on diet foods. They will know how to observe their pets for changes in the courses of diseases, and tend to consult you more often. They will often ask you for services such as blood tests, radiography and ultrasound without you having to do a selling job.

Pets belonging to these well-informed clients opting for a high level of veterinary attention will reap the benefits. They will be healthier, have their problems diagnosed earlier and lead more comfortable lives.

You as the veterinary surgeon will enjoy a far greater degree of job satisfaction when dealing with high quality clients. It is easy to treat everything in the same way, not to tax yourself by explaining anything and to keep dispensing the same tablets. Stories abound of old-style vets (all now long gone, I am sure) who worked in a consulting room with just one bottle of yellow injection (antibiotic) and another of clear injection (steroid) – or in one more sophisticated case I heard of, a ready mixed bottle of the two – and ready dispensed packs of red pills, white pills and black and red capsules. Simple, efficient, profitable but somewhat lacking in skill or ambition I tend to feel. How much better to actually make a diagnosis, to know what sort of tumour you have removed, to visualise that endocardiosis which you can hear through your stethoscope. When starting out in practice everything seems exciting (sometimes in the same way as a roller coaster is exciting) but once you have mastered the basics, you need to exercise your mind to keep sharp and to be at your best.

Methods of client education

With the best will in the world, of the torrent of information which you will be keen to pour out to clients in your consultations, very little is likely to stick. I know this because it is common for clients, after I have spent a period discussing the possible side affects of treatment, to call the practice and complain that the dog is drinking to excess (because it had a diuretic?) or is very sleepy (acepromazine?) or has a hole in it (been spayed?). Have you ever got lost in a large town or an out-of-the-way corner of the country and asked a local for directions? Being very familiar with the locality, the helpful person will probably give you excellent and detailed instructions, most of which you will forget as soon as you wind up the window. To get directions that you can follow, you are better off asking someone who is familiar with the area but doesn't know every piece of pavement or tree. Clients are in a similar position when they come to see you. You undoubtedly know your stuff (I'm trusting you here), but can you transmit the information which you want your client to retain in a suitable fashion?

I would suggest keeping the details that you tell the clients simple. Make sure that they grasp the salient points. Make sure they know that you know far more about the condition or the treatment than you are passing on, since they need to know that you are in control, but give them mainly the information which is necessary for them to know what is wrong, and what the rationale behind treatment is. For further detail, make use of the printed word. This can apply to all aspects of contact with clients, from diseases to routine health care, from worming to information about operations. Don't rely on the client remembering all the information which you tell them, after all they are not taking notes and there are often more interesting things than you at the clinic to claim their attention.

These are some of the areas where the printed word is useful.

Newsletters

These are an excellent way of communication with clients. We produce four newsletters a year, which are available at the practice and are sent out with booster reminders.

Each newsletter contains one or two longer articles about a disorder or a topical subject. There is a section with the latest practice news, about staff, events or new equipment. We usually include reminders about worming, weight clinics, old age check ups and a variety of other services available at the clinic. Occasionally adverts for drugs or foods are scanned in. A cartoon or two is included. An interesting case history may be inserted, or pictures of cute patients. There have even been vouchers printed, for reduced-price microchip implantation for example.

The newsletter serves as a useful client education tool, a gentle form of advertising and a reminder that we offer a wider range of services that the average client may not be aware of.

My own feeling is that it is far preferable to produce your own newsletter in house. There are some generic newsletters which I have seen offered which practices can customise, but they seem to be of pretty poor quality, and inevitably can't give an impression of exactly what your practice has to offer. They have to deal in general terms with topics in case they describe facilities that some practices do not provide. Far more personal to do your own thing. With a computer and a photocopier it is relatively easy and quite satisfying. Most vets are capable of writing interesting short articles, and if you run short of inspiration you can always make use of drug companies' material or data from one of many internet sites. Create a template which will be used as the basis for each issue. Two to four sides of A4 is a convenient length. Ask around the practice staff for volunteer contributors. Many vets, nurses and receptionists can turn out very tidy articles.

Once you have produced the newsletter, make sure that it is distributed widely. You will find that it is popular and gets clients asking you about services, rather than you having to introduce the subject.

Handouts

A library of handouts on various disorders is very useful. They enable you to educate clients about whatever their pet happens to be suffering from, familiarise them with the treatment and any alternatives, and let them know what the likely prognosis is. They can also be produced to describe the reasons for neutering, information about operations, worm life cycles, general information about puppy healthcare and training and a variety of other subjects. As well as informing clients, they perform the useful function of standardising the practice approach to dealing with various problems and the advice given about routine healthcare. They save the vets much time and answer many questions which clients would probably want to ask when they get home.

Here again I feel that it is better to produce in-house information sheets. Drug manufacturers produce many leaflets and flyers, but although often excellent they do appear rather like brochures or advertising, which of course they are. By all means lift the information that you want from these sheets, but a handout clearly prepared by the practice will seem more like an information source and any recommendations for treatment will seem much more impartial.

Have a standard template for the handouts, and keep them to one or two sides of A4. Make sure that they are easily comprehensible to the lay person. Have a supply copied and ready for dispensing with treatment.

The waiting room

As your clients wait to see you or your colleagues, they might as well be subjected to a little gentle advertising. Make use of eye-catching and informative posters. Ensure that they are rotated on a regular basis. Posters should ideally be presented in frames, and tatty older ones should be thrown out.

Notice boards are very useful education tools. Keep them neat and tidy, and use them for displays about various diseases, worming, fleas, puppy education. Nurses are often happy to be given the job of notice board maintenance, and can be quite inventive when it comes to displays. Make use of manufacturers publicity material, but take the scissors to it and produce the display that you want.

Pre-operative instructions

When booking patients for surgery, give the owners a sheet of instructions on pre-operative preparation. Note the date and time of admission, feeding and watering instructions, notes about emptying bowels and bladder before arriving at the surgery, suggestions about any extras the client may want performed (nails, teeth, dematting) and information on pre-operative health tests. You may also give notes about when the patient is likely to go home, what food it is going to be allowed that evening and what the owner should expect.

These pre-op sheets prove a great help, and greatly increase the uptake in blood tests and ecg's, which we all like to perform, but don't necessarily like to be seen as selling.

Consent forms

I'm sure that all practices use consent forms, but do make the most of them. Here again sections allowing clients to request extra procedures or pre-op tests should be included. A note about the possibility of anything going wrong should be on the page. Take contact numbers for the client which will be relevant during the day.

The correct use of consent forms is important. For them to be meaningful the client must understand what he or she is signing. Avoid using shorthand or abbreviations (even GA should be written out in full). Be specific when describing what procedures are to be performed. If you are unsure of all that will need doing, write down 'and further treatment as necessary' or similar, and get the client to agree this. Ensure that the client reads the form before signing. Don't let the client sign without reading; if they have forgotten their glasses, read the form to them.

Post-operative instructions

As a client collects their pet after surgery, they will firstly be in a state of high excitement, pleased that their pet has actually survived your ministrations, and then in a state of shock as they write out the cheque to pay for your valuable services. They are in an even less suitable state than normal for fact retention, so make your discharge sheets as informative as possible. Give information about feeding, exercise, wound care and what to expect from the pet. Describe what you have done, the results of any pre-op tests, any further tests that you recommend, what treatment you have prescribed and what the next steps will be. We include a section telling the owner what parasites we have managed to turn up while examining the patient.

A separate post-op sheet for dentals is a good idea. We include a dental chart, a description of what we have done (useful to demonstrate that they are actually good value), and details on preventative home dental care.

In this way you should avoid those phone calls asking why Simba has a large shaved area around his wound, or why he has a shaved area on his leg without a wound, or why he has still got a scrotum when you have castrated him.

Vaccination health checks

There is a common tendency amongst the public to fail to appreciate the full value of the annual booster visit. To them, the visit consists of a linger in the waiting room, a few pleasantries with the vet, an injection, and a parting with some cash at the reception desk while the staff try to sell them wormers, flea treatment and all sorts of exotic food.

This is not a satisfactory state of affairs: partly because they should appreciate the importance of the health check that their pet has received and partly because, if they are not going to appreciate the work that you have put in, you feel as if you have wasted your time and the temptation must creep in to do exactly what they assume you have done – vaccinate the pet and no more. Many clients will miss the fact that you have been examining their pet, so efficient have you been. Many clients have minds so occupied with other things that they even miss the fact that the vet has already injected their pet, and there is an awkward silence while they wonder when he is going to get around to it, and the vet wonders why they are still there. Make your clients appreciate this annual visit. Emphasise in the booster reminder literature that this is a vaccination and health check. Point out to them that if it is indeed true that there are seven dog or cat years for every human year, then a yearly check for their pet is only the equivalent of a visit to the doctor every seven years for ourselves.

Most useful, however, is a sheet which very briefly details the organ systems which you have examined, any problems found, and what action is advised. We include the weight of the pet, together with an ideal weight, and advice on worming and flea treatment. This will bring home to even the most oblivious of clients that you have been doing something to earn your money. It also serves as a persistent reminder of the advice you have given regarding dental treatment, dealing with lumps and bumps or any other suggestions which they can normally conveniently pretend not to have heard.

Action plans

If your practice holds weight clinics, geriatric clinics or similar, be sure to have clear written instructions to give to clients to help them follow through any advice they have been given. They can digest the information given at their leisure. If you have made the therapy sound inviting, then they are more likely to take it up. Weight charts and score charts for symptoms such as arthritis are useful aids.

Using the media

The general public is to a large extent animal-mad. They love programmes about animals and stories about animals in the press. They follow news stories about animal-related subjects. They also seem to pay much more attention to what they see or hear in the media than they do when a mere 'real' person deals with them. One of my clients came in to a consultation in a high state of excitement, claiming to have seen a condition shown on a veterinary television program which she was sure her tubby, bald dog was suffering from. Hypothyroidism, she pronounced with great satisfaction. This would have been very useful, were it not for the fact that the lady in question had paid for a series of blood tests, had the results explained to her (as I thought) and was presently complaining about the difficulty of stuffing several thyroxine tablets down her dog's throat daily. Sometimes I feel that if I really want to get a point across I should videotape myself and give the tape to the client so that they can hear the information from a trustworthy source – the television.

On the other hand, real-life veterinary programmes can be very useful. They often highlight a variety of disease conditions which owners can then identify in their pets, and rush them in to the practice to have their home diagnosis confirmed. This reduces the need for you to convince them of the need for treatment as this has already been done for you. In fact many pets greatly benefit from this increased awareness of clients, and we have had quite a few serious ailments presented to us much earlier than they otherwise would have been.

Make full use of media examples to demonstrate or illustrate diseases and symptoms to your clients. They will make your life much easier if you take advantage of them. It does, however become necessary for you to sit and watch these programmes, or read the latest stories in the press. Apart from the normal run-of-the-mill disorders which are covered, there will be occasional scares or topical subjects. It never ceases to amaze me how even a tiny snippet hidden away on page 14 of a newspaper will bring a torrent of enquiries. Be prepared to answer any concerns that such stories raise.

Value for money

Successfully getting your message across to clients will give you satisfaction, will convince the client that you know what you are talking about and allow them to understand your treatment regimes, and will hopefully ensure that the pet receives the right care from you and its owner. One of the most useful aspects of good communication is reassuring the client that they are getting good value for money. Veterinary care is undoubtedly expensive these days. We know that compared to many other services, including the medical profession, it provides amazing value for money, but if we are to be able to charge realistically it is vital that the clientele know this as well. Telling them what we do and ensuring that they understand it is the best way of doing this.

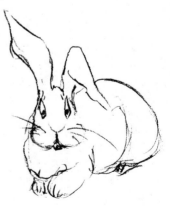

- Misunderstandings are some of the commonest causes for complaints and second opinions
- Don't assume that clients understand what you are saying
- Avoid jargon
- Good efficient history taking is one of a practitioner's most important skills
- Clients who understand you complain less, feel involved and allow you to do more
- Make use of handouts and newsletters to get your message across
- Practice forms should be clear, informative and helpful
- Consent forms are worthless if not filled in correctly and understood by clients
- Use television, newspapers, magazines and books to help illustrate your points

4

Clients have pets as well

Pets are loved

With all the efforts being expended in caring for clients it might be possible to slightly neglect the feelings of our animal patients. This would be a mistake as people genuinely are quite potty about their pets. One occasion on which this was brought home to me involved an out-of-hours call late one evening. The client needed to be seen urgently because her guinea pig had fallen down two flights of stairs. I arranged to see her at the surgery and drove in muttering to myself about the possible reasons a guinea pig would have for negotiating stairs at eleven o'clock at night. In due course the client's car arrived. She emerged from the driver's side. The other door opened, and after a slight delay, her husband gingerly extracted himself from the passenger seat. He hobbled towards me doubled over like some overdone caricature of Richard III, occasionally emitting a low moan. He

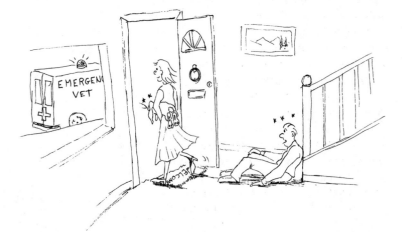

was cradling something with one arm. When they entered the clinic, all was made clear. The husband had in fact been holding the guinea pig while *he* fell down two flights of stairs. While he looked rather the worse for wear, the guinea pig had obviously been comfortably cushioned and looked absolutely fine. When I had reassured them as to its state of health, they thanked me and disappeared off in the direction of the local casualty ward to have the poor man's injuries tended to, happy to do this now that they knew the guinea pig was safe and sound.

Pets really are child substitutes, but frequently appear to be held in higher regard than people's children. The fact that they are unable to speak up for themselves seems to heighten an owner's sense of responsibility. They feel any ill treatment or pain that their pet suffers almost more than the pet does. We forget to care for these little darlings at our peril, for although clients may be prepared to put up with some deficiencies in our handling of humans, they won't tolerate our taking their pet's feelings for granted.

Whatever a human may think of you and your practice, if their pet is keen to visit the clinic, they will be too. It grieves me when we occasionally have a client who, having dragged their reluctant dog across the waiting room floor, polishing it nicely with the pet's bottom, then says 'It must be terrible when none of your patients want to see you. Just like us and the dentist, eh?'. 'No! No! NO!' I want to shout. 'Your dog is the only one today who is the least bit circumspect about us and our consulting room.' Most of them have to be restrained from queue barging. While their owners have a chat and become so engrossed in local gossip that they almost forget why they are sitting in this comfortable building, the dogs all await every opening of the consulting room door with bated breath, salivating in their excitement, straining at the leash in their eagerness to be the next to enter. When they hear their names called, they bound forward, hauling their human baggage with them. Pets have enjoyed visiting the clinic so much that not only do we have a steady stream of cats and dogs who trot along to us if they have become lost, but some of them actively break out so that they can come and join us. One beefy boxer used to regularly leap out of his garden and hare along several streets to the surgery, where he would scratch and whine at the door until he gained admittance. The fact that he started doing this after he had visited us to be castrated also provides a useful

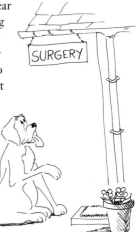

piece of evidence for owners (usually male) who feel that this procedure is the most psychologically damaging act that we can perform.

I feel that I am in a fortunate position, in that I am able to indulge my love of animals and have many animal friends while conducting my chosen profession. If we can transmit this to our clients, they will have far more trust in us than they would if we simply demonstrated a formidable level of veterinary skill and knowledge, but no feeling for their pets.

The first time

The first consultation with a puppy or kitten is a vital one. You, as the stranger, are at a slight disadvantage here. The young pets are usually brought in to see us within a day or so of leaving the security of the litter. They may or may not be appreciating the care and love they are receiving in their new home, but they probably won't be appreciating the fact that they have been subjected to a car journey and a whole new set of frightening smells and noises and dumped on your consulting table. If things are not well planned, they will be briefly and clinically checked over, having various previously private orifices explored and cold hard objects stuck into unmentionable areas. Their reward for this is to have a sharp needle full of some icy cold fluid rammed into their neck, and to be dropped back into a dark box, smelling strongly of the vomit they produced in the car on the way over. This is an experience that is likely to scar a kitten or puppy of even the strongest character.

We are all aware now of the importance of the early socialisation period in a cat or dog's life. Their experiences in the first few weeks of life will shape their view of the world for the rest of their lives. We must be absolutely sure that we give them a good impression of us and our place of work. I prefer a kitten or puppy to have a visit to the surgery which doesn't involve pain before we start assaulting them. Accordingly we offer a free puppy or kitten check, at which time we can get to know the pet a little, carry out our clinical examination and make a fuss of the pet. This saves time a few days later, when the vaccination course can begin, as you won't need to give a thorough check, but just go over any points raised at the first visit. We always make time to fuss a pet, if their nature allows, whatever the age of the pet. Often the pet is greeted before we start on the client. This shouldn't be a perfunctory pat, but a reassuring greeting, stroke and general admiring of the pet. Make the pet at ease before finding out its problems. Be gentle on handling. Do all you can to gain the pet's friendship and confidence.

To make our lives easier, we encourage the animal's new owners to use the socialisation period to get the pet used to the practice environment. This is easier, and more important, with puppies than with kittens. Get the owners to bring in puppies regularly, whether to meet staff, be weighed or just to sit in the waiting room. The range of pets and experiences that the pup will encounter will be of great use to the owner. What a great place to see dogs of all shapes, sizes and temperaments, cats, birds and a gamut of human beings. We also ask owners to spend time each day examining their pet's mouth, ears and paws. We make them do this until the pets are quite relaxed about having these areas felt, looked at and held. If the owners are willing and capable, they can be encouraged to clip a little off the claws on a regular basis, thus hopefully averting the traditional sense of panic and fear of torture that this process seems to induce in even the most placid of pets.

The combination of fuss, treats and familiarity should produce a mentally well-balanced pet which sees the practice as just another fun place to visit, filled with well-meaning humans who find them irresistible, which is just as it should be.

We tend to also spend extra time on those adult pets who are visiting the clinic for the first time. Many of these will be apprehensive of veterinary surgeries either because of unsympathetic handling, or because of a painful or frightening experience. As you are a new environment for them, you have the chance to regain their confidence. Dogs and cats are not stupid. They know full well that this is a veterinary surgery, and that the person with the crocodile smile and the green or white coat is probably bent on doing them physical harm. They won't be one hundred per cent sure, however, since everything is that much different, so make the most of your window of opportunity. Show them that vets can be fun! If you succeed, you will steal a march on the previous practice, which will do you no harm, even if it is rather unfair on your predecessors.

Calming techniques

It is our good luck to be presented with a variety of different species to practice on. All of these are capable of becoming upset in their own little ways. Working out how to calm and reassure pets eases our work and keeps clients happier. Stressed pets are remarkably good at hiding even the most severe of symptoms. I sometimes wonder whether I shouldn't make more use of adrenaline as a front line drug. The number of times a dog which has been unable to use one or more legs (even had broken legs) has undergone a remarkable cure just by being presented in my clinic are legion. Sick birds unable to raise a chirp sing their little hearts out when they see me coming. Dogs and cats which we have been called to because the time has come for euthanasia can be seen running hell for leather round the garden, or doing the wall of death (apologies for the term) round the living room as we contemplate holding this creature still long enough to administer the *coup de grâce*.

To get a real idea of an animal's state of health you should examine it in a resting state. Ideally we would see them in their home environment. Although this is necessary for some exotic species, it is not practical for many of the pets brought to us. We therefore need to allow them to relax and show their true status.

Begin by watching them in the consulting room. Observe them at rest and when walking to your room. Once in the room reassure them and relax them if possible.

Dogs, cats and several other species respond well to a gentle voice and a steady stream of reassuring, quiet chat. This is one of the things I found a little difficult to master as a new graduate. Inevitably there is a certain degree of self-consciousness about a young vet, trying to look at his professional best, talking to a cat or a budgie. Does one carry on a normal conversation, as though one expects the pet to understand every word? Does one use baby talk or strange cooing noises? Is there any chance that one will be taken seriously whichever course of action one takes? Don't worry. With time you will become quite inured to the embarrassment potential. In most cases you are in the presence of the pet lover, where normal standards of behaviour and mental state are suspended. It doesn't matter what you say to the pet. One of Shakespeare's sonnets or Scene 2 of the *Texas Chainsaw Massacre* are all the same to the creature as long as the delivery is right. So take the opportunity to flatter and butter up the pet, by which I mean the client. Tell it how handsome and clever it is, how well-proportioned and well-behaved. Just as clients take it personally if you tell them that their pet is obese, they also feel that any compliments paid to their pets are by rights shared with them. There is nothing wrong with this; make use of it. I once saw a young bitch who was a regular and sweet visitor. When I had finished and was waiting for the client to leave, she stood there looking rather disappointed. In reply to my enquiry, she said that Pebbles was upset because I hadn't called her darling as was my normal practice.

Just as stroking a pet is therapeutic for humans, so the animals also get a positive effect from gentle, smooth contact. Dogs and cats in particular feel the benefit. Hand-reared parrots also tend to appreciate stroking or scratching, as long as you can deliver this in a calm way, i.e. you are not so scared that the bird can detect your terror. Do think, though, before dishing out cuddles to all and sundry. Species not used to being in contact with humans will become more stressed if constantly handled. This may not be apparent as they may simply freeze. You will be thinking that you have a wonderful touch as you have persuaded this baby wild rabbit or tiny finch to sit so beautifully still, whereas the animal is simply highly stressed and may even succumb, taking their final revenge on you by dying. This will happen to you at some stage in your career, so be prepared, and if you have to handle highly-strung pets, warn the owners of the possible effects.

Try to encourage a calm atmosphere in the surgery. If the waiting room and reception are bedlam, your patients won't be all that calm when they come to see you. If practical, shift noisy and boisterous dogs away from cats and meeker animals. Put your child control measures into action if someone's little darlings are poking into all the cages and counting Rottweiler's teeth. Exotics being particularly prone to stress, see if you can accommodate them in a quiet room or area, or schedule birds' appointments, for instance at a quiet time of day. If you are busy and in a rush, try not to communicate this to your patients. Don't use this as an excuse to be brusque and rush the examination.

Clients are often in a highly excitable state when they come to see you. They are worried about their pet, they are worrying about their next appointment somewhere else, they are worrying about the bill. Pets being highly attuned to and taking their lead from the owner's state of mind, will be similarly worked up if they have an owner like this. You know all those 'pet which looks most like their owner' competitions? If they ran 'pet whose character most accurately reflects their owner's' competitions, many people would be in for an eye-opening. Time and time again we see that neurotic pets belong to neurotic owners, calm pets to calm owners, and outgoing friendly pets to outgoing and friendly owners. Many clients seek behavioural and chemical cures for their pets' psychological problems, when if they could only sort their own problems out the pets would be fine. It isn't your job to treat owners, or even to tell them this, unless you happen to have degrees in subtlety, charm and psychology. You can however recognise the symptoms and try to gently steer the pets in the right direction. Difficult, stressed or aggressive pets in these circumstances are often better parted from their owners when you come to examine or treat them. Without their pack leader to take a cue from and gain confidence from, they are often easier to handle. Don't always be in a rush to lift middle to large-sized dogs onto your consulting table. The unfamiliar sensation can seriously add to their stress and might make them aggressive. Come down to their level to help relax them.

Birds are a group of species which I often separate from their owners for examination and treatment. This is partly to reduce the transmitted stress as described above. It is also sensible for any stressful procedures to be performed by strangers, as birds will for ever more associate their owners with a fearful or unpleasant experience if they are involved in it. Far better for us strangers to be the nasty guys and not to damage the owner-bird bond. Another reason for handling birds ourselves is that owners are so awfully bad at it. This applies to cats and dogs as well, where the advice of some professional indemnity insurers is to have a qualified member of staff doing all the handling, but it is particularly true of bird, and especially parrot, owners. The owner's idea of restraint falls sadly short of our requirements for safety of handler and vet, and comfort of the bird. If owners are allowed to handle the parrots, someone is likely to get hurt, hopefully the owner, although in these litigious days a bite from a macaw may seem a mere kiss compared to a solicitor's bite. You need to see these animals in the course of your work. My best advice is to become familiar with them and the methods of restraint, and to have at least one member of staff who is happy to assist you and competent at handling. The fact that one can catch and safely restrain a parrot is enough to qualify one as an avian expert in many people's eyes.

Birds are best initially examined in a darkened room, where they will be naturally calmer. For your ease, when you come to catch them up, they should be at a level below your shoulders, so that they are not in a position of dominance. A nightmare situation is the owner who walks in doing a Long John Silver impersonation with Polly on his shoulder. The bird is in a prime position of dominance close to its spiritual leader, and it isn't going to give up this position without a fight, which will often involve Polly's well known impersonation of a ticket punch with the client's ear taking the less popular role of ticket. Parrots should also be at or above waist height or they will become too stressed, which in birds in particular is potentially disastrous. In these days of safe isoflurane anaesthesia, it is quite legitimate and even desirable in many cases to briefly anaesthetise an avian patient to allow detailed examination and administration of drugs without stressing the patient. Always explain to the client if this is going to be your course of action. Although often the safest route for the bird, it is still important to point out the possible dangers of anaesthesia.

When restraining birds, and again parrots in particular, a towel is far superior to gloves. This is partly because the towel is more effective, and safer for bird and handler, but more importantly because birds are very shape conscious. Consequently they will become hand-shy if caught with gloves, which is not likely to endear you to the client. Along similar lines, the owner-bird bond is going to be severely tested if the client has to administer treatment of various types on a daily basis. Fortunately, although birds can remember the shape of a face very well, they are hopeless at seeing through disguises. Advising the client to wear a hat, a bag over their head (do explain why if you want to keep the client) or a Halloween mask (no, the bird won't be scared by it) will be enough to stop the avian patient from associating its owner with this tormentor. There are some advantages to being bird-brained.

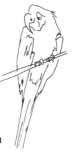

Reptiles will also form a part of your workload. Many vets are even less familiar with these strange beasts than they are with birds. One would hope that clients who had taken it upon themselves to own reptiles would be familiar with their care and handling. Sadly, in these days of pet supermarkets anybody who walks in off the street can take a lizard or snake home and install it in a little glass prison. For all the shop knows the entire extent of the knowledge that the purchaser has about his chosen species is that he saw a picture of one in the *National Geographic*. It never ceases to amaze me that pet superstores self-righteously trumpet their policy of never selling puppies or kittens on grounds of welfare. Let's face it: although the sale of puppies and kittens is not morally pleasing, dogs and cats are very easy to keep. People have to be almost wilfully ignorant to induce severe ill health in them, although they do. Most reptiles and amphibians, however, are highly demanding in terms of diet and environment. In well over 90% of cases, to sell these animals is to condemn them to a long slow death. Only the fact that they have such a slow metabolism enables them to stay alive for such a long time.

In one respect, this widespread ignorance of their acquisitions' requirements, together with an inability to reproduce them, means that you automatically know what is wrong with every sick reptile that is brought to you, and most 'healthy' ones. Owners mistake the ability to stay alive for health. I doubt that many captive reptiles are truly healthy. Thirty years ago pet shops everywhere had pens stuffed full of tortoises. People would buy them for a few shillings. These creatures are capable of living for well over a hundred years if given the faintest chance. With such a life span, if every tortoise ever sold in this country had lived we would have wall-to-wall tortoises in this country. You wouldn't be able to walk from your front door to your garden gate without tripping over a dozen of the pesky chelonians. We do have a few tortoises still going strong now, but these belong to people who have by skill or luck, combined with a very adaptable tortoise, managed to provide roughly the right conditions. Even then, several forty or fifty year old tortoises are really just being unconscionably slow in dying, living on unsuitable food and deprived of all but a fraction of the quantity and intensity of sunshine they evolved to enjoy. There are over 700 known species of gecko. Many of those offered for sale or even displayed in zoological collections can't be positively identified. Each of those species has evolved to live in a certain environment. Reptiles just are not adaptable like mammals, and to a certain extent birds, are: ask the dinosaurs. If we don't even know what the species is, how can we possibly know what to offer it in terms of shelter, nutrition, temperature, humidity and any other secret ingredients?

You may gather that I feel that the handling of these poor creatures is the least of their concerns, but we do owe it to them not to make their lives any more miserable. My point, made in a somewhat long-winded way, is that the owners are unlikely to be skilled in the handling and restraint of their pet. For the purposes of allowing examination it is fine to allow the reptiles' body temperature to drop, which will induce a state of torpor and allow easier examination. If you are to administer any sedatives, anaesthetics or drugs, however, remember that it is unsafe to keep the reptiles out of their normal temperature range, because of the severe effects on their ability to metabolise such chemicals. Point out to owners as well that reptiles need to be at the top end of their temperature range to ensure a working immune system, whereas the pathogens affecting them are quite happy at a lower temperature. Be firm but not rough when holding reptiles. Snakes are prone to bruising if handled too tightly, and the bruises may develop into abscesses. Many lizards are in a state of poor calcium balance, and may either already have pathological fractures of their limbs, or be about to receive some as you try to control their flailing legs. Dark, soft cotton bags are useful for placing both snakes and lizards in to keep them subdued at the surgery. Iguanas will often be calmed if you cover the 'third eye', or pineal, on their foreheads.

Small furry creatures often present quite a challenge in handling ability, never mind calming skills. Hamsters, mice and gerbils will be good if regularly handled by their owners, but many are left to their own devices for long periods, a state of affairs they seem keen to prolong. They certainly don't take kindly to a vet grasping them and prodding them. My best advice here is to be brave if bitten. Many of us have hurled a hamster across the consulting room in a reflex action designed by the body to rid itself of a painful object attached to a finger, and definitely not designed to endear us to the poor six year old watching wide-eyed as her pet describes a graceful arc through the air. This is probably not the time to remind the client of the worrying news clipping about the policeman who went round to a family to reassure them after some minor crime. Things were going well and he felt that he was doing a good job of liasing with the public. After enjoying a cup of tea and patting the two young boys on the head, he moved towards the door. As he walked, he felt a ball roll up against his leg, and playfully kicked it towards the two lads at the other end of the corridor. It was only as it crunched against the far wall between two deeply shocked faces that he realised he had just propelled the family hamster in its exercise ball a good five yards down the hall.

Rabbits and guinea pigs can be in a state of terror so deep that they freeze when examined. Don't fool yourself that this is a result of your calming influence or some rabbit hypnosis technique. Rather try to reduce any extra stress and keep your handling of animals thus affected to the minimum. These pets are rather less likely to drop dead in your hands than small birds, but massive adrenaline levels are not going to improve their condition.

Rabbits and rats are very often labouring with severely compromised lung capacity due to chronic pneumonic lesions. Even if the owners haven't brought them in for a respiratory complaint, watch them closely for signs of respiratory distress. It will do your reputation little good to cause respiratory or cardiac failure in your patient.

Avoiding further stress

Even if we have proved very successful in our welcome to pets and our gentle handling procedures, we have to accept that many pets are going to be a little apprehensive at seeing us in the surgery. They are in a situation where a human other than their beloved pack leader is taking awful liberties with them, looking in areas which are really rather private, and inserting objects into areas which are really rather unmentionable. We don't want to reinforce this apprehension and fear response by unsympathetic treatment. By defusing their worries we should be able to get them to accept their journeys to see us as merely an interesting diversion. A little thought and sympathy on our part can remove many of the more painful or unpleasant stimuli that pets are subjected to.

It may seem a small matter, but injection technique is of great importance. Let's face it – the vast majority of visits to the vet are going to end with the sadist in the white coat inserting a shining metal pin with a horribly sharp end into some part of the pet's anatomy. Make the experience as painless as you can, and that is one less thing for the pet (and owner) to worry about next time round. I take great pride when I am told that I must have a gentle touch as Poochy didn't seem to feel a thing. I also take it as a challenge when I am told that a pet doesn't like injections and will make an awful fuss. Most of our canine patients, due to gentle injecting and a little judicious bribery, prick up their ears and become quite animated when they hear the wrapper coming off the syringe. When a client has more than one dog I sometimes have to fight them off as they both eagerly try to get to the front of the queue.

Firstly, use the smallest gauge needle that is practical for the drug which you are injecting. For all free flowing drugs I tend to use a 25 gauge needle, even in dogs. We keep 27 gauge needles for our exotic patients. Particularly for puppies and kittens having their vaccinations, I tend to draw up the vaccines with one needle, which could be an elephant needle if it makes things quicker, and replace the blunted needle with a fresh 25 gauge one. In this way there is almost no pain.

Distraction is an important part of the process. I know that my brain is capable of really concentrating on one thing at once. For me that might involve doing the crossword while listening to music – either I don't hear the music or I fail to complete the crossword (which, of course, I normally succeed in doing). For the patient it means that a loud voice talking to them and reassuring them reduces their sensitivity to the pain of the needle. Just as my mother used to believe that a firm blow to the good leg always made a sore knee seem much better, a firm grip and vigorous rubbing of the scruff slightly away from the injection site often completely distracts the patient. After injecting, more vigorous petting has a similar effect, while the owner thinks you are just being very friendly to the pet. In one of my clinics, my practice budgie, Paxo, used to do the honours for cats being anaesthetised. He sat by the prep room table and fascinated the cats to such an extent that few of them even realised they were being rendered unconscious. Finally, for dogs a treat tends to work wonders. Most Labradors are rendered almost brain dead by the offer of a titbit, and all sensation seems to disappear.

Be sympathetic in your drug selection, and choice of injection site. When giving puppies their inoculations, remember that vaccines removed from the fridge are cold. Warm the vials by rolling them in your hands for a minute. This can be done while you pass on a few gems of wisdom to the client, so no time is wasted. Clients always marvel at how well pets accept injections, comparing them with their own experiences. In part this is because the medical profession seem to delight in rummaging around for the largest bore, longest needle they can find before administering the jab. Mainly, however, it is because animals are blessed with a scruff, and don't need to have their muscle fibres stretched apart by whatever drug is being inserted, causing a regiment of pain receptors to fire at will. Take advantage of this piece of luck. Use the scruff if an intramuscular injection isn't indicated. After a few weeks in practice, most of us will be aware of the injectable drugs which sting when used. It is a bit sad when the pet accepts the injection without a murmur, then starts to rush about the room trying to claw at its neck, or worse still sets up a plaintiff, piercing wailing calculated to wither the confidence of every pet in the waiting room, and sending the owners pale. If you can avoid the painful ones, do so. There is often an alternative, or even no real need for the injection. This may again seem like the simplest of advice, but I wouldn't include it if it wasn't frequently ignored. The blind use of the 'correct' drug regardless of the patient's feelings is rather cruel if not necessary. It also becomes firmly imprinted in the pet's mind, which will give you problems in the future.

Injections are not the only procedures which cause stress to our patients. Claw clipping and ear cleaning or examining are famous examples. How is it that such a simple, and hopefully pain-free, procedure as claw clipping can turn the mildest mannered dog into a rabid monster? It is a long time since I first saw practice as a schoolboy, but the most vivid memories that I have are of a succession of snarling, growling, struggling, biting poodles and terriers who had come in to have their nails cut. I am sure that there were other cases, but none of them seemed to involve the personal dangers that pedicure entailed.

To achieve these procedures calmly may well take quite some ground preparation. Whenever young dogs come to see you, whatever the cause, get them used to you holding their paws and peering into their ears, so that they appreciate that this isn't necessarily a painful process. You may even do some totally unnecessary claw clipping so that you only need to take the smallest nibbles off, and the dogs understand that its quite comfortable. Give them plenty of praise afterwards, and many of them will shrug and think 'Hey, if that's all it take to please you, clip away'. When you do have to deal with painful ears, force yourself to be gentle and reassuring. The owners are going to have to continue the treatment at home, and the last thing that you want is to have the whole process develop into a twice daily battle between owners and pet. If the ears look extremely sore, explore the possibility with the owners of having the patient in for a quick anaesthetic to allow proper examination and cleaning. If this isn't on the cards, give a couple of days treatment before trying to poke your auriscope to the end of the horizontal canal. I know that the theory states that you should examine the status of the ear drum before commencing therapy etc., but if that ear is really sore, inflamed, thickened and filled with debris, you are not going to see anything like an eardrum down there. Think of the patient.

Try to avoid too many heroics in forcing pets to accept treatment. I know that it has to be done sometimes, and we have to force the pets to submit for their own good. I've done it, often. Whenever I am forced to use strong arm tactics I do so with a heavy heart, knowing that my relationship with that pet is going to be the poorer for it. If pets have had a particularly nasty experience, either at your hands, or in an incident outside the surgery, bear in mind the useful amnesiac properties of diazepam. These are effective on events that occur soon before the dose of the drug, and may well blot out the unpleasant memories.

Chemical aids to animal handling

We do have an array of artificial aids to help us in our dealings with pets. I have mentioned the benefits of a strategic dose of diazepam to help obliterate unpleasant memories. Experiment with other drugs and chemicals to see if they will help ease your patients' worries.

Tranquillizers are readily available for use. Used sensibly they will make events more pleasant for you, the pet and the owner. Give tablets for owners to use before the pet arrives. Use tranquillizer and analgesic combinations on pets once at the surgery if they are worked up or upset. Far better to use a chemical restraint on a fractious dog even to clip its claws, rather than to cause it physical and mental anguish.

A thorough examination of birds, especially those unused to handling, is often only achievable by a quick anaesthetic. If well used, this reduces the stress for the pet, allows a proper exam. and the collection of blood or other samples. The benefits of stress avoidance and detailed examination should well outweigh the risks of anaesthesia, assuming that you are sensible in your use of the procedure.

Don't forget those prickly little balls of mystery, hedgehogs. There are several paragraphs and many pictures of methods of unrolling hedgehogs for examination. Forget them. Even if they work they tend to result in the hedgehog rolling up again with your finger firmly trapped like a sausage in a spiky roll. Isoflurane and hedgehogs go well together, and they may actually get some relevant treatment as a result.

A recent development is the introduction of preparations containing cat pheromones. Originally introduced as an aid to the treatment of spraying, they are useful for calming cats and making them feel secure. I would advise owners of nervous cats to try spraying their cat baskets with them for more relaxed travel. A few judicious squirts in the consulting room introduces a friendly atmosphere for the feline patient. Using the scent in hospitalisation cages helps reduce stress and is quite helpful in aiding recovery by producing happier cats. There is a variety of the preparation designed for helping to calm fractious cats. There may be further developments in this field, and they are worth watching.

Bribery

I have mentioned the use of treats when injecting pets as a part of the distraction process. We also have used treats for many years as a reward for good behaviour, a pleasant introduction to the clinic, or a compensation after having something unpleasant done. My own spaniel desperately volunteers to have her anal sacs expressed or to receive an injection so that she can have her reward. Many of our canine patients are similarly obsessed. I see that many practices now use this little reward system, which is good news for our patients. When we started doing it, though, it was quite a novelty, and impressed clients greatly.

Start off with puppies when they first come in, whether or not they are having any treatment at that time. They are not so suspicious as older dogs and will usually accept treats in the spirit in which they are offered. Many older dogs clearly think that they need to be on their guard all the time, and suspect that I may be trying to slip them a poison pill. Once puppies have got the idea that free grub is on offer, they tend to remember this even if they only visit once a year.

The treats that we use are vitamin pills, which have the added advantage of showing clients how tasty they are, and maybe making a sale. At one time in the past, when the treats I was using weren't being accepted as often as I would have liked, I resorted to buying a huge tuck shop bottle filled with white chocolate buttons. These were accepted with enthusiasm by even the most reticent patients. I did, however, seem to go through the jars rather rapidly. Only when I caught my nurses with their hands in the jar, so to speak, was the mystery cleared up. Since then I tend to stick to treats which are more attractive to pets than humans.

Although dogs are the most susceptible to bribery, it is worth experimenting with other species. I find that I can usually get kittens to accept a broken-up vitamin tablet, which not only distracts them as I give then their vaccinations, but helps to keep them on the table rather than wandering around the consulting room. Ferrets find a vitamin and malt fish flavoured gel produced for nutritional support of sick cats quite irresistible. They will lick at a dollop of this gel stuck on the table while you examine and inject them, quite oblivious. My only worry is that they are so keen on it that they might consider my finger, with the odour of the gel on it, as a more substantial snack.

Finally, don't forget your human customers, particularly the little ones. A few rewards for children won't go amiss, although they may go missing if your nurses have a sweet tooth.

Outside the consulting room

Clients who see us outside of our normal environment, and out of our working uniforms, often have trouble in placing us. They are sure that they know us, but are not quite sure who we are. Their pets suffer no such problems. One sniff and they know exactly who this sneakily disguised human is, and depending on your relationship with them, they will act accordingly. There was a pleasant pub which I used to frequent. From the first time that I went in and sat at the bar, and every time subsequently, the two corpulent Boxers which lived there used to take up position on either side of me, and bark incessantly. They never made an aggressive move, and were in fact quite prepared for me to stroke and fuss them, but they obviously saw it as their duty to warn all animals in the neighbourhood that the vet was in town. The landlord swore that they never did this to anyone else, and the strange thing was that they weren't even patients of mine, at least not to begin with. In the end I opted for quieter surroundings if I wanted refreshment.

If we can persuade our patients that we are just normal friendly people worthy of their acquaintance rather than white- or green-coated sadists, it will greatly help our relationship with them once through the consulting room door. One place to cultivate the relationship is outside of the consulting room. Welcome pets to the practice. Make them feel like popular guests. Dogs are suckers for a bit of flattery. Encourage the owners to bring them in when they are not in need of treatment, so that they can get used to the practice and the staff. Give them a treat and make a fuss of them.

Puppy parties are a great help in establishing the practice as a place of fun and socialisation for dogs, rather than a frightening place where they have to behave perfectly and are rewarded by thermometers up bottoms and needles in scruffs. For participants, the clinic will be another pleasant excursion, just like the park, the woods and Auntie Flo's.

If you have dogs of your own you will come into contact with clients and pets at exercise, at training classes and at shows. Take every opportunity to worm your way into their affections.

Staff involvement

Ensure that all the staff are involved in the campaign to befriend patients and set them at ease. Veterinary staff are usually only too happy to fuss pets and compliment them. Let them know that this is to be encouraged, together with the strategic use of treats. Get them to use their initiative in making friends with pets, both inside and outside the practice.

It helps to have staff who keep a variety of breeds and species, and who take part in showing, dog training, agility or any of the animal-based recreational activities. This helps to bond with clients, and lends more weight to advice given.

Experience of keeping pets

Without owning pets, it is hard to really empathise with your clients. It is possible to know the theory and the right advice to give, sure enough. What is hard is to appreciate the difficulties involved in looking after an animal, the pleasures they give, the frustrations they cause and the heartache when they become ill or die. You must have a pet to realise how hard it is to get a tablet down one, how difficult it is to rest one or keep it indoors, how long it really takes to bathe one, why brushing cats' teeth isn't the most popular of pastimes. You need to keep an animal to understand why owners can't remember to treat for fleas regularly, mislay their vaccination cards and still have half their antibiotic tablets left when they should have been used up days ago.

When you are a pet owner you can discuss problems with clients from a position of shared knowledge. You are better placed to understand their difficulties and to pass on tips for getting around them. Owners will have more faith in your advice if you can show them that you have been through the same experiences. If you have fed a range of foods, or used five different flea treatments, they will take your advice because not only do you know what's right, but you have tried it as well. When prescribing treatment, you will take into consideration not only what is theoretically best for this patient, but also what is going to be easiest practically for the owner and pet to cope with.

It is helpful not just to keep pets, but to keep, or have experience of looking after, a range of pets. Small furries, birds, fish and reptiles are very different, and bring a whole host of separate practical problems with them. The practicalities of something like tortoise hibernation are far easier to deal with if you have been through the experience yourself. Your advice on house training rabbits and avoiding multiple appliance failure as they chew their way around the house will carry far more weight if you have worked things out at home.

Clients naturally will lend more weight to advice from a fellow enthusiast. This is evident from the way that your advice rarely carries more weight than that of a breeder, a pet shop owner or a friend who 'used to keep one of these'. Once they know that you have owned a cockatoo or a snake or a tarantula the value of your opinion will be elevated to the same lofty level as the opinions of these other worthies. If you are unable to keep every type of creature, a common problem, use your staff's experiences. Between all the members of staff at a practice you should be able to amass a considerable amount of knowledge of different species and breeds.

Know your species

Just as keeping a range of creatures is useful, it is important to have a reasonable depth of knowledge about the species which you will see. For clients to take you seriously, you should know, for instance, the way to tell a male budgie or cockatiel from a female. You should be familiar with the more common species of exotic pets which you will see, so that you can recognise them. You will also need to know their dietary and environmental requirements.

A wide range of creatures are kept as pets, and it is not possible to know all about every one. I have seen at different times the entire UK population of a species of duck, and snakes and geckos which have been unidentifiable as far as the dealers who sold them were concerned. What you do need, if you are to be taken seriously, is a knowledge of those species which can be considered common, and a set of good reference books to back up your knowledge. Where birds, reptiles, fish and invertebrates are concerned, good texts on their natural history and biology are more useful than veterinary textbooks, as you will often find the answer to their problems in their management.

- Don't spend so much time keeping your clients happy that you neglect their pets
- If a pet enjoys your practice, its owner will as well
- Make visits a positive experience for puppies and kittens
- Be proficient in handling and calming the whole range of species which you will treat
- Don't aggravate a pet's illness by unnecessary stress
- Think about avoiding inflicting pain on patients
- Bribery is good
- Everyone in the practice should welcome pets
- Experience of keeping different species is invaluable

5

The art of persuasion

The need for persuasion

Sometimes clients can be the most frustrating creatures. You may spend a good few minutes explaining their pet's problems, laying out a sensible course of action and be on the point of making all necessary arrangements when they will turn around and say that they would rather not have the treatment, the operation or the investigations. They have a certain reluctance to commit their pets to tests or surgery. There is an abhorrence of medications which must be given 'for the rest of his life'. There is an irrational (to us) fear of anaesthetics, of steroids, of antibiotics, of vaccines or any of a hundred drugs and procedures. The reasons for their reluctance may stem from worries about the side effects of treatment on their pet, to worries about the side effects of treatment on their wallets, to an irrational (to us) wish to spare their pets unnecessary suffering. They will often say that they don't want to put their pet through the danger or discomfort of surgery, thereby implying that they are happy to leave the large ulcerated and infected tumour *in situ*, or to leave the pet with terminal halitosis and such large accumulations of tartar that it cannot close its mouth properly, or that the dog can probably manage quite well even if its leg is fractured in three separate places.

Such misconceptions and well meaning reluctance for treatment are damaging not only to practice turnover, but to the pets' well being. We have a duty to ensure the comfort and health of our patients in spite of their owners' desires. Although we can't go against an owner's wishes, we can gently work to persuade them that we have got their pet's best interests at heart and are not simply trying to swell the practice coffers while taking the opportunity to carry out surgical experiments or medical trials using their pet as a guinea pig (even if it happens to be one).

In many ways we work in a difficult age when we have a constant need to justify our decisions and actions. Times were when if the vet or doctor said that something needed doing, then it was done. Nowadays there is always some television programme, or newspaper article or internet site which has an opinion to offer. Vets have to present a good case for their advice if it is to be accepted. In some ways this is good, as it ensures that we really are sure of our ground, but it can prove rather wearing. The problem is worsened by the media's love of a good scare story. They whip up a storm about some procedure or medication, milk it for all it's worth and then move on, leaving us to clear up the fall-out. The modern suspicion of all things which are not 'natural' is a problem as well. Owners are often more willing to accept a 'natural' treatment than a medicine, even though the medicine has to be shown to be safe and efficacious, whereas there is no such requirement for 'natural' remedies. In my opinion this lays clients open to making considerable outlays on ineffective remedies. They are willing to continue with these even if they see little improvement ('because you wouldn't expect a dramatic effect') and even though the pet is deriving no benefit.

While not wishing to be blinkered in our approach (I would expect vets to be open-minded about all proposed therapy, and to examine the actual evidence), we often will have to encourage owners to see the light, while at the same time not appearing to be mercenary and insensitive. Not always an easy task.

In using persuasion to encourage clients, we must steer clear of coercion. It would be possible to bully clients round to your way of thinking, but beware the possible consequences. Ours is an imprecise art. We can't guarantee that events will go according to plan when dealing with living organisms. Even the most simple and innocuous treatments and medications may induce an unwanted reaction in the patient. We cannot be expected to predict this, but the client will still expect us to do so. If you have forced a client against their will to follow the path which has led to the complication, then you will find it all the harder to extricate yourself from the situation without shouldering all the blame. The right to grant consent must lie with the client, and only in exceptional circumstances when the well-being of the pet is severely threatened should you ride roughshod over that right.

Advantages of keeping pets

We have discussed the benefits of keeping animals so that clients know that you are familiar with the joys and frustrations of pet ownership. So much easier to persuade someone to try various avenues of healthcare if you and your menagerie have been down that road already, experiencing the benefits and the difficulties en route. When Mrs Sceptic looks you in the eye and says 'So you find clipping your cat's claws weekly and brushing its teeth every other day a breeze, do you?' you can look right back and reassure her that this is so.

I think that it is important for you to appreciate the anguish involved in making decisions about your own pet so that you can sympathise with your clients and understand why they appear to be so blinkered on occasion. You need to understand why they are reluctant to take the risk of a life-improving surgery, even though to your mind there is no shadow of a doubt that operating is the right thing to do. You should be concerned about the use of vaccines or insecticides or processed food on your animals, and if you rationally decide to go ahead with such treatments, then you can feel confident in your advice to clients.

The 'my pet/my friend' approach

The average person feels far more confident in making a decision if someone has been there before him; made the mistakes, discovered the hidden problems and reaped the benefits. This is why we avidly devour consumer reviews and seek the opinion of someone who has already bought a Sinclair C5 before we go out and part with our hard-earned cash. Consequently, you will find it easier to steer clients along the path which you have chosen for them and their pet if you can cite examples which you have personal experience of to illustrate your point.

The most effective persuader is the 'my pet' approach. 'My bitch had a

mammary lump appear last year
and I had no hesitation in performing surgery. She's fine
and healthy now.' For a bit
of extra drama you might
add that your (less sensible) friend had a bitch,
ignored the small mass in
the caudal mammary
gland, and the next thing
she knew the bitch had secon-
daries in the lungs. Be careful how much
you use this ploy, or your clients will think that you have the
most unhealthy, accident-prone bunch of pets in Britain. It is an effective
approach, especially if true. Clients will often ask you what you would do
if the pet in question were yours. This is a great opportunity to give them
the hard sell, but I tend to be rather reticent. I will say what I would do,
but I also point out that I have the opportunity to do everything I can, and
I won't be faced with such a large bill at the end of the day.

If you can cite the example of a friend who has had a pet with similar
problems to those of the client's animal, this will also be a big persuasion
factor. Try to be honest, but a little embroidery is useful to allow a full pre-
sentation of the possible outcomes following a course of action. You might
mention a friend whose dog underwent an aural ablation and describe one
or two of the possible post-op complications and how the friend coped
with them. You can certainly point out the improvement in the dog's aural
health and comfort, and how long it took to resolve. You might use the
example to hint that longer-term treatment of the remaining horizontal
canal may be needed on a long term basis. Be imaginative with your example.

The next layer of persuasion by familiarity is the database of clients you
have who have followed the therapy you are recommending. We have a list
of willing volunteers who own pets which have lost limbs, or undergone
aural surgery or chemotherapy, and who are willing to speak to clients
making the decisions on these matters for their pets. It is very reassuring
for a worried client to hear how someone else has coped, and maybe to see
the animal in question. These clients are a great help to us and usually tip
the balance in our favour. I try to get them not only to point out how wonderful life is for the pet now that they have fully recovered, but also to go
through the worst aspects of the procedure and the aftercare, so that the
clients about to experience this for themselves can be reassured that they
can cope.

The soft sell

One of the hardest aspects of our profession is the need to charge for our services. It hangs over me whenever I am giving out advice, painfully aware that what I suggest is going to cost money. Some vets are consummate masters of this financial aspect, but many feel that they are being viewed as salesman, that the fact that the practice will be paid for our work taints our advice.

We must learn to cope with these feelings if we are to be successful. Like it or not, practices must earn money. We shouldn't feel guilty for being paid to do our job, just as all our clients are undoubtedly paid for theirs. You must give the best advice as you see it. Don't feel bad about selling a complete flea treatment regime with effective and safe remedies. If the clients don't buy the treatment from you they will get it from a pet shop, using chemicals with poorer efficacy and safety than you can provide. If you feel that certain blood tests are indicated and helpful, advise the client accordingly. They can always decide not to follow your advice. Theirs is the decision to spend the money. A common mistake that we as a profession are often guilty of is that of trying to save or spend the client's money. It is up to them and not you to decide whether they can afford what you are advising. Clients are usually surprisingly willing to spend their money on the tests and procedures that we advise. By trying to save them money you are doing your practice a disservice and you may be denying clients the right to have the treatment that they would want for their pets. So don't try to dissuade clients from procedures which you think may or may not be helpful. Present them with the facts, tell them how much it all will cost and let them decide.

Although we needn't feel bad about taking money for our services, I feel that we shouldn't be seen to be aggressive in our selling techniques. Don't force the client to buy this or to have that done. Let them make the decision. I am a bit dubious about special offers and campaigns to get clients to buy the latest drug. The drug companies will like this approach, trying to get all cases of dermatitis onto the one antibiotic. Buy 50 boxes of this drug, then work hard to pass it onto the clients. Rather than base your advice on whichever shelf in the pharmacy happens to be most overloaded, follow your clinical judgement.

One more point to remember about charging is that the main item that we have to make money on is our time. Try to educate clients away from the idea that they are paying for drugs and other items. If they aware that the bulk of what they pay is for your time and advice, you will find it easier to charge for consultations. If pets are always given an injection and drugs to make it easier to justify charges, then when they have a consultation which merely involves giving advice, and you can't think of any drug which you can actually justify dispensing, clients may find it hard to see why they should pay. Have the confidence in your worth and the value of your time to charge properly for it. In any case, if you dish out free advice, and some other professional charges forty or fifty pounds for their advice, the client will perceive the expensive advice to be of more value. After all, as everybody knows, 'you gets what you pays for'.

Examples of situations needing persuasion

The following are just some of the common areas where you may find clients wavering or questioning the need for a course of action. No one can provide the easy answers for dealing with these situations, but it is helpful for you to be aware of them and to work out your own strategies for dealing with them as they arise, and they will.

Vaccinations

Annual booster vaccinations are a hot topic at present. The public is fed a series of scare stories by the media, who like to seize upon a controversial topic and work it for all its worth, before dropping it and moving on to the next disaster. The problem is that although many clients retain a healthy scepticism when reading such stories, the seeds of doubt are planted in their mind and you are the person who is going to have to reassure them that it is both safe and necessary to have their pets vaccinated. Media scare stories don't always work against us. The same papers which now happily suggest a list of evils which may befall dogs receiving vaccinations were only too pleased to fill their pages with horror stories of parvo virus epidemics when the disease first showed itself. Those stories resulted in queues down the streets outside veterinary surgeries as anxious clients rushed to get their dogs vaccinated. (It's a pity that there wasn't a specific vaccine available at that time.) The impact of such stories is far reaching. Even though the original epidemics were decades ago, many clients are only aware that their dog receives a parvo jab, and are ignorant of the other useful components of the vaccine.

My approach to clients who worry about the safety of vaccines is not to dismiss the extremely dubious evidence quoted out of hand. After all, we are not omniscient and it is always possible that adverse effects of vaccines will be discovered. There are already one or two cases where they are implicated in disease: post-vaccination sarcomas and the discovery of distemper virus inclusion bodies in some bone cells in a few cases of hypertrophic osteoarthropathy for instance. I do explain that there is at present little sound evidence to show that annual vaccinations are implicated in diseases. The fact that a disease occurs in a vaccinated animal isn't proof. Try demonstrating to them that, for example, 70% of dogs with fractured femurs were vaccinated within the previous twelve months. Anyone can see that this doesn't lead to the conclusion that vaccinations cause fractured femurs (hopefully). Have the results of any studies that have been done on the subject to hand. Explain that it is easy to start a rumour, but to substantiate it with scientific proof is not so simple.

I then cover the undoubted benefits of vaccinations. How they have improved the life expectancy of cats, dogs and rabbits dramatically. Point out how many puppies and kittens used to die unnecessarily from parvo, distemper and feline enteritis. I also tell them about cases of the diseases involved which we have seen at the clinic in recent times. I will also stress that Leptospirosis is a zoonosis.

Clients must make up their own minds about the benefits or perils of vaccinations, but we should ensure that they have facts rather than hearsay to base their decision upon. We in turn should be open-minded and keep up to date with developments in this field, although at present I belong to the camp which can see many benefits and few dangers. We can't deny that vaccinations are an important portion of practice revenue, but we can easily survive without them. It would simply be a case of charging realistically for other procedures at present subsidised by boosters, and keeping a large isolation ward for the regular stream of patients with messy diseases.

Health checks

One of the major benefits to the pet of an annual vaccination is the health check that they receive at the same time. It is an excellent opportunity to assess an animal's physical and mental condition and to dispense appropriate advice to the clients. They can be kept up to date with developments in the veterinary field, such as new theories on feeding, training, parasite control and care of chronic disorders. Clients can be spectacularly unaware of changes in their pets' health status, and it is almost necessary in many cases for a vet to examine them so that abnormalities are detected.

When pets are brought for their annual boosters, there is no problem in ensuring that they receive regular examination. It is when the owners have opted not to continue with boosters, or when pets are older and you feel that they would benefit from more frequent routine checks that you may need to sell the idea to the clients. Again, those on regular medication are easy to persuade. They appreciate that the condition being treated needs to be monitored, and it is your decision how often they are seen. If the pet is healthy, a client may need a touch more persuasion. Make use of practice newsletters and literature to stress the importance of the health check.

Point out the wide range of conditions which you might be able to detect on these visits, and how much more effective treatment is likely to be if instigated early in the course of a disease. By the time that a client detects a symptom, a disease may be so far advanced that you can only offer palliative treatment. Clients will often ask you whether it's true that there are seven dog or cat years to one human year. My advice is to agree that this is so, and therefore a yearly check at the veterinary clinic equates to a visit once every seven years to the doctor's surgery. Once the pet is a geriatric, surely they can see that a 'yearly' or 'biannual' visit to ensure that diseases of old age are picked up early on would be advantageous. Another useful approach is the 'dentist' one. Most of our pet patients have teeth, and their owners are used to the idea of a twice yearly dental check. Since pets' teeth are usually in a worse state than ours, it is not too hard to persuade clients of the need for a regular examination of their dentition.

Laboratory tests

There are still some older members of our profession who chunter on about how the younger generation of vets is unable to make a diagnosis without using a laboratory test, how the art of veterinary science is dying and how they managed to diagnose and treat their patients with only their hands, a thermometer and a stethoscope to help them. Absolute poppycock. What they really mean is that they didn't have a clue what was wrong with their patients, and fortunately a proportion improved with the treatment meted out to them, while others with 'incurable conditions' declined rapidly or slowly. I can see the huge difference, just in the time that I have been practising, that the laboratory back-up we have now has made to our detection of disorders and our ability to treat them. In days gone by a cat which drank a bit more than normal had kidney failure, and a coughing dog had 'heart disease'. When I first started work, disorders like hyperthyroidism and pancreatitis in cats and dust-mite allergy or Addison's disease in dogs were considered almost unheard of. Without in-house laboratory facilities and with senior veterinary surgeons frowning on the sending-off of samples we all too often failed to recognise the conditions which we were dealing with. How much better for our morale and job satisfaction, and for our patients' well-being that we now have such tremendous facilities available to us.

It is my experience that rather than having to persuade clients to opt for blood tests, x-rays and ultrasound examinations and other forms of investigation, it is the vets who need to be prompted to carry out these tests. This stems from a reluctance to spend the client's money, a reluctance to perform tests if one is unsure that they will confirm one's tentative diagnosis, or sometimes an overconfidence in that tentative diagnosis. To deal with these matters one at a time, it is not up to us to save our clients' money for them. To do so is fraught with possible pitfalls. We may be denying a client the best attention simply because they look poor. We may be badly misjudging their financial situation, and so not only doing them a disservice but unnecessarily denying the practice funds. Often, the clients turn out to have pet health insurance, and our sense of self-congratulation at shaving a few pounds off the bill can melt into a puddle of disappointment. Worse still, if we delay an accurate diagnosis and effective treatment by procrastinating on the appropriate investigations, we may be costing our client more and even laying ourselves open to action.

The reluctance to perform tests until one is sure that they will confirm one's suspicions is an interesting scenario, although all too common. If one is absolutely sure of the problem, why do the test? Surely it is when one isn't sure of the problem that the investigations are most useful. Clients understand this, and they are not going to be disappointed if the results are normal. That is good news, remember? Having said that, even if one is pretty sure of the disorder being dealt with, it is comforting to have confirmation, and useful to have a measurement of how advanced the disease is. Don't be too confident that you are right in your supposition until the proof is there for all to see.

Clients are used to investigations being performed when something isn't right through their own experiences and through watching medical dramas on television. They are usually pleasantly surprised by the cost of such investigations, so I feel that perhaps it doesn't take too much persuasion in the majority of cases to allow you to use investigative procedures. You can even impress them hugely by providing them with the results and an interpretation within a day, when they are used to a wait of weeks to find out what has been found on an x-ray or blood test on themselves.

If you feel investigations are indicated and clients are reluctant, explain the potential savings from an early diagnosis. Show them how an accurate diagnosis will guide the therapy and management of the case, and give an idea of the prognosis. If you are discussing routine health checks for pre-operative cases or geriatrics, demonstrate how laboratory tests are able to pick up early signs of organ failure long before a physical examination can. In pre-operative checks this may avoid serious complications or even save the pet's life. For geriatrics, the early instigation of treatment for organ failure will bring the most benefit.

Diets – weight reducing and clinical

Many vets find it hard to commit themselves wholeheartedly to selling diet foods to clients. They may feel that pushing certain foods in this way is crossing the pet shop line. Consequently many pets are denied the benefits of an important aid to the treatment of their diseases, because although the correct diets are mentioned, they are done so in passing or in a half-hearted way. In fact, it is often hard to provide the correct balanced diet for a specific disorder by using a home-cooked diet, or modifying the normal food that a pet eats. The very soft sell approach which many vets are fond of, where the correct feeding is discussed with a few options mentioned, and the client is left to make their own decision, is not very effective. Clients may be full of good intentions to help their pets, but once out of the surgery other things take priority. It is also easier for them to believe in a product if you show that you have confidence in it. This means deciding what you consider to be the best diet, and recommending that alone.

The following are some of the areas where clinical diets benefit pets, and some ideas for clients to mull over.

Obesity is a perennial problem. A consequence of nutritious food, insufficient exercise and a misguided desire to spoil the pet are to blame. Even getting people to recognise that a pet is overweight is difficult. Many a Springer spaniel with a back broad enough to lay out tea for eight has walked in (often accompanied by an owner who looks as though he has consumed tea for eight) with the owner completely oblivious of the fact that his pet is not the normal shape for the breed. On seeing the weight of his dog, compared to the breed average, he may pass some comment such as 'Well, she's always been a large one', or 'She's big boned', or the favourite excuse 'Well she's been spayed, hasn't she?'. Many clients prefer to have their dogs or cats a little rotund, and are horrified to see a truly fit pet, suspecting the owners of gross negligence. The fact that obese pets often belong to obese owners is an awkward one to overcome, and somewhat cramps your style when handing out the dire health warnings and strict diet advice.

I don't need to point out to you the many adverse effects on health of obesity. There are few conditions that are improved by being obese, although I have had a couple of large dogs which were possibly spared more serious injuries when involved in car accidents because of their extra padding. We make use of a handout which contains the reasons why obesity is not good, records the starting and ideal weights and has a chart on which to plot the anticipated reduction in weight. We put plenty of encouraging statements on the sheet, pointing out the most common reasons for weight gain, and debunking the common excuses.

It should be possible in almost all cases to lose weight without the aid of prescription diet foods, but there are some pets which stubbornly refuse to lose weight while their ration is shrinking to painfully small dimensions. The anguish of the owners is hard to bear. Eventually, there is a worry that in order to restrict calories sufficiently we are depriving the pet of sufficient quantities of other vital nutrients in the food. Here a prescription food is inevitable. In most cases, however, the prescription food will bring about a more rapid loss of weight, encouraging the owners to persevere, and allowing the pet to eat a little more bulk than if their normal food was simply fed in tiny portions. By encouraging your clients to bring their pets every two weeks to be weighed and have their progress discussed, you can confirm in your mind and theirs that the diet is worthwhile.

Chronic renal failure was one of the first conditions for which clinical diets were developed, and it remains a disorder which is greatly improved by dietary therapy. In recent times our knowledge of the factors involved in the disease has led to improvements in the diets, and more reasons why a home-cooked diet just isn't as good. It is actually quite hard to produce a home-cooked diet which fulfils the criteria of correct protein quantity and quality, sufficient energy to maintain weight and a good balance of vitamins and minerals. Most important of all, current thinking suggests that a low phosphorus diet is valuable not only to alleviate the symptoms of renal failure, but also to slow the progression of the disease. The old 'white meat diet' which has been a standard piece of advice for 90% of pet disorders, just can't deliver a low enough percentage of phosphorus. In any case, most clients would soon become fed up with the chore of preparing a special recipe food for their pet each day. Most, if persuaded of the need for dietary manipulation, would rather do it the easy way.

Hepatic disorders, diabetes mellitus and *urolithiasis* are some other conditions where dietary therapy is either valuable or indispensable. Once again, convincing the owners of the benefits of clinical diets shouldn't be too hard as long as time is taken to explain the mechanisms of the diseases and exactly how the diets work. Simply giving an owner half a dozen tins of food and saying that that is the food to use is unlikely to inspire much commitment on the client's behalf. Make use of your own back-up literature and the manufacturer's material. All the diet food manufacturers are only too happy to provide plenty of interesting-looking leaflets which explain the mode of action of their foods. You must provide some input as well to lend credibility to the literature. Be comfortable selling these products secure in the knowledge that you are helping your patients and, by reducing the need for other treatments, you are also helping the owners.

Operations

There is a great fear of anaesthetics amongst the public which we, being all too familiar with the procedures, tend to forget or ignore. Something which to us is a quick and routine procedure, such as a cat spay or a general anaesthetic for an x-ray, is a very stressful experience for the owner. In fact, out of the owner, the vet and the pet, it is the owner who will be the most bothered by the whole process. This, to us, irrational fear is used as a justification for leaving an animal in discomfort or for laying it open to further, potentially lethal, consequences, particularly if the pet is aged. In order that we can ensure that our patients are allowed the benefits that the procedures we wish to perform will bring, we may need to practice our powers of persuasion and reassurance.

We have a slightly difficult task here. We should never be blasé about the possible dangers of general anaesthesia. If you are in practice you will experience 'unexplained' anaesthetic deaths. They are not only devastating for owners, but extremely emotionally traumatic for the veterinary staff involved. Murphy's law dictates that if anything is to go wrong, it will be when you have an owner who was very concerned about the anaesthetic to begin with, and whom you possibly had to cajole into allowing you to proceed. So, however hard you are working to encourage the surgery, don't make the mistake of promising that it is risk-free. Far better to compare the infinitesimal risk that the general anaesthetic carries with the far greater risk, or even eventual certainty of death, that not proceeding brings. Be honest, and allow that accidents can happen, but quote the safety record of the practice, the precautions taken to prevent such an accident and the great increase in safety that modern anaesthetic drugs and regimes bring.

Dental treatment and wound suturing are two examples of procedures which clients often ask to be performed without general anaesthesia. It shouldn't be too hard to convince them that the stress involved in restraining and treating the pet, allied to the discomfort that they feel, makes anaesthesia the best option. Point out that although possible to conduct the treatment without a general anaesthetic, it is not possible to do such a good job, and there would be a severe compromising of the quality of treatment.

Although it can make practice staff rather nervous, I rarely use age as an excuse not to treat a surgical condition. A cat of 18 years of age with a tumour might have two or three years of life left if it is treated, and a small tumour may be easy to remove in an eighteen year old cat, but a large tumour in a nineteen year old cat will definitely have increased complications. Having left the tumour, however, it may have grown to proportions which dictate that we either operate or opt for euthanasia. Tumours and bad teeth won't get better if ignored. Far better to grasp the nettle and treat at the earliest opportunity. Some clients find it a consolation if they are assured that once asleep there is no distress to the pet. Even if they were to succumb under the anaesthetic, it would be no different to being euthanased.

Clients' concern over the safety of the anaesthetic process allows you to recommend the use of pre-anaesthetic health checks. Performing a bio-chemistry profile and haematology, together with an ecg will help to put their mind at rest, give you added confidence, and is a useful source of practice income. I am not being commercially callous here, but the use of laboratory equipment for pre-anaesthetic testing lets the equipment earn its keep, allowing the practice to invest in better quality resources than it could otherwise afford. On occasions in a young pet these tests may show up an undiagnosed problem which wasn't suspected. Be warned, however. Because of the range of results which will be found in a population of nor-mal animals, statistically, some results will fall outside the quoted 'normal' ranges. The more tests performed, the more likely a rogue, 'abnormal' result is to show up. Thus if you perform a 12 test profile on a healthy ani-mal, it is likely that one of the results will fall outside the normal range. Be sensible in your interpretation, but also be ready to explain this to the client. In older patients, I consider pre-operative testing to be invaluable. With the benefit of hindsight, it is possible to recall cases of apparently healthy pets which came in for routine treatments such as dentals or minor surgery, made uneventful recoveries and then went down with kidney fail-ure a few days later. Pre-anaesthetic testing would have revealed compensated chronic renal disease in these individuals and allowed appro-priate preventative action to be taken.

Be honest, be persuasive and don't let irrational fears or ageism deprive your patients of the treatment you feel that they need.

Treatment for less valuable pets

Exotic species are a problem for many practices. In the past, clients have often been charged very little for their treatment, partly because of the low perceived value of the creatures, and partly because the practitioners may have felt that their limited knowledge reduced the value of the service being provided. We still charge considerably less to treat 'children's pets' than we do for dogs and cats, but our prices are gradually becoming more realistic. They have to as these creatures demand just as much time as larg-er ones, and they often involve far more of the veterinary surgeon's time in research and devising therapy. Some exotic creatures are worth far more than the average dog or cat and are charged accordingly, but their owners are usually only too happy to pay for treatment. Rabbits have graduated from children's pets to the substitute child status that their canine and feline equivalents enjoy. There is still, however, a hesitation to seek treat-ment for the hamsters, mice and budgies of this world.

I am always rather taken aback when a client asks how much a course of treatment for a small furry will cost 'because it only cost four pounds', implying that it would be far cheaper to simply get a new one. My replies vary according to my mood and audience. For one thing, I point out that children can be obtained free of charge, but that they are usually considered worth spending money on. I will remind the client of their responsibility to any animal that they decide to take on. They may not ignore its discomfiture simply because it is cheap to replace. The very least that they are obliged to do is to choose euthanasia rather than continued suffering, although if they take this option when treatment is available they are not responsible enough to get themselves a replacement.

On the other hand, it is as well for us to be aware that the average client will baulk at paying too much for their small pet's treatment. We should aim to give value for money and not to introduce unnecessary costs. Be knowledgeable and confident to reassure the client that they are receiving a level of expertise equivalent to that which a dog or cat owner will get. Know your client as well. Some are positively keen for you to exercise all your clinical skills regardless of cost. Good communication is the key. Often a client who seems very reluctant to spend money on their child's pet is pleasantly surprised when given an estimate of the cost involved, having expected a sum much higher.

Treatment for the ailments of old age

Ageing pets are all too often the victims of quite unintentional neglect and cruelty by their owners. This is not to say that they are unloved, but there is a tendency amongst clients to dismiss the symptoms of many geriatric disorders as simply 'old age'. It can be hard to persuade clients that there is no such disease as 'old age', and that all the symptoms they see are coming from specific disease entities, which may be more common in older individuals, but are not an inevitable consequence of ageing. Thus it may be seen as acceptable for an old pet to limp, to be covered in lumps and bumps, to have a poor smelly coat, to have appalling dental disease, to have chronic diarrhoea or incontinence, to show symptoms of senility, to have sticky, pussy eyes, to have chronic otitis externa, to cough, to be unable to exercise or to be sick once a day. We must be careful not to reinforce this callous attitude by agreeing that a problem is 'to be expected at that age' whether because we fear it may be hard to treat the disorder or because we haven't the energy to persuade the owner that something can be done.

Your mission, should you choose to accept it, is twofold. Firstly you must make clients aware that their pet actually has a problem, and secondly you have to make them see that the problem can be treated and that it is worthwhile to do so.

Often the first time that a geriatric disorder is presented is when the pet is brought for its annual booster. Either the client will mention a symptom, such as lameness, as an afterthought or in a reluctant way, as though they don't want you to say that you can help, or you will notice the symptom and point it out to the owner. This is fine, but many older pets don't come for boosters, and in any case a year is a long time for a geriatric patient. Plenty can happen to a dog between the ages of twelve and thirteen, for instance. Increase your clients' awareness of the need for more frequent checks in older animals by publicity campaigns in the waiting room, or articles in the practice newsletter, or mailshots. Consider holding geriatric clinics and sending out invitations to owners of older animals. Have an extra value price for a geriatric health check, including blood tests and ecg.

Most clients have no intention of being unkind to their pets, and once they realise that there is a treatable condition to be dealt with, they will be willing to try and improve their pet's lot. Offer them effective remedies and be sure that they have realistic expectations. You are dealing with chronically damaged organs here which may not regain full function. Your aim is to improve function as far as possible and to relieve discomfort. Once they see a little improvement in their pets' condition, clients will be enthusiastic about continuing therapy, and will probably spread the word to other owners of senior citizen pets.

Dental care

Here's an interesting contrast between people's perception of their pets and themselves. Many pet owners will go on and on about how they love their animals, they would do *anything* for them, and they definitely don't want them in discomfort. Many of them will also chunter on about how awful their own dental problems are. 'I can take any sort of pain, until my teeth are involved.' You know the sort of thing. Those self-same people are often happy to ignore the severe dental disease that their pets are suffering from. Sometimes they are simply unaware that there is a problem, no doubt considering it normal for their pet to smell like a rotting corpse and for odd teeth and bits of calculus to drop out of the pets' mouths from time to time. Others simply don't seem to consider it important. You may lift the dog's lip during a routine examination, and after recovering from the involuntary recoil and donning a pair of gloves, you show the owner what he's been missing. The owners then shrug, say 'Oh dear' and mildly agree that the mouth has seen better days. You can see that they have little intention of doing anything about it.

Dental disease is something that will affect at least 80% of our patients (canine and feline). Probably more if they live long enough. It isn't simply cosmetic, but a serious health hazard in terms of pain, stress, malnutrition and local and haematogenous spread of infection. Here is an opportunity not only to provide a steady practice income, but also to seriously improve the lot of your patients.

I believe that most clients who ignore their pets' dental problems are either genuinely unaware that bad teeth cause a problem, or are reluctant to put their pets through an anaesthetic just to have their teeth cleaned. You can reassure them as to the safety of anaesthetics and educate them as to the wide range of secondary disorders that poor teeth lead to. Take every opportunity to examine pets' teeth, whatever else they come in for. Have a dental health handout which reinforces the points that you are making, and perhaps have a score from zero to five for the sake of their pet's teeth which you can fill in so that they are aware of where they stand. Many owners seem full of good intentions while they are in the surgery, but their resolution evaporates as they leave the front door. If you haven't persuaded them to book in their pet there and then, then having a hard copy reminder will at least jog their memory. Make use of all the practice publicity avenues to raise awareness of dental disease.

Home dental care is another much neglected area. To be fair, clients these days are far more likely to wield the toothbrush than in recent times, when it was simply a big joke to even consider brushing pets' teeth. Start educating clients when their pets are young. Far easier to get a pet to accept interference with its mouth when it is youthful and thinks that everything done to it must be normal. This is also the time when clients are devoting most interest to their pets and so more likely to try these wacky ideas out. Far harder to start when the pet is eight, knows its mind and has sore gums anyway.

Choose your clients well when advising on home dental care. We have a whole range of products available to us now ranging from toothpaste and brushes, through technical chews to plaque control foods. Don't be too dogmatic. We know that brushing is the best form of home care, but it is far better to use an easy method which will be performed daily, rather than choosing brushing if it is done once a fortnight or only for the first few days. Be sympathetic as well. Try the methods out on your own pets. If you are able to brush your cat's teeth successfully, congratulations. You may advise your clients accordingly with a clear conscience. I have to be a little more circumspect and admit that I use methods which involve less use of martial arts and more guile. Ensure that your clients' expectations are realistic. Home care won't eliminate dental disease. I always point out that although I brush twice daily and use the dreaded floss, my hygienist still finds plenty of scale to scrape away every six months. However you choose to proceed, try not to become bored with dental disease and join your clients in dismissing it as being of minor importance. It is important and deserves our best attention.

Insurance

Pet insurance is one of the great liberators for vets in practice. Statistics show that the average bill for the treatment of an insured pet is around 25% more than for an uninsured one. As the insurance companies appreciate, this is not because of an unethical bumping up of the bill for those that can afford it. Rather it is a consequence of the wider range of tests and more sophisticated treatment that a vet feels able to use on an insured animal. Our in-built reluctance to spend our clients' money is to blame. I wouldn't say that we fail to provide a proper level of service to the uninsured pet, but it is a different level of service. Before I am shouted down by a howl of protest, the statistics speak for themselves.

Clients are not always quick to pick up on the benefits of health insurance. They receive 'free' medical attention from the NHS, although nothing is free, and the actual contribution they are paying via taxes and National Insurance is quite high. They tend to be optimistic as to the pet's chances of leading a healthy and fit life. They are also under the misapprehension that the excess claimed by the companies refers to each and every visit to the surgery, rather than to the whole course of treatment.

Although we don't directly benefit materially from the recommending of insurance, in terms of commission, we do get the advantage of being able to perform our job more thoroughly. I feel that it is well worth our while advising clients to consider insurance. The rash of new companies trying to muscle into this field presents a new set of difficulties. Many of the new policies sound very tempting in terms of premiums, but turn out to offer very limited cover or cover for a very short period, or to be draconian in their exclusions. We cannot be expected to be familiar with the details of every insurance policy, so I would advise a practice to choose one or perhaps two companies that they are happy with, and to stick to recommending their policies. This gives the clients more confidence as well. They are more likely to follow your advice if you are offering them one policy which you are happy with, rather than vaguely recommending insurance and supplying them with a bundle of leaflets to go through.

Paying bills (getting your money)

Vets are again in an awkward situation when it comes to the financial side of our transactions, complicated by our natural wish to divorce the clinical and cash sides of practice. For some reason we are cast as the bad guys if we show reluctance to treat a case, never mind that the client has no money and no prospect of paying, and that their neglect has caused the suffering of the pet. Oh no, once the problem is laid at our doorstep, it is our moral responsibility to sort things out. Well, no one should expect us or our staff to work for nothing. Never lose sight of the fact that you are a professional selling your services, not giving them away. You are entitled to be paid for your work, just as the client is entitled to be paid if he decided to work. How would your average client feel if his boss said 'By the way, I'm a bit short of cash this month, but I can pay you ten pounds now and I'll bring you five pounds a fortnight until we're straight.' I can just imagine the response. Don't be made to feel guilty for doing your job.

Some clients will expect as a matter of right to be able to purchase a service or some treatment, such as flea treatment, and be allowed to walk out with a promise to pay the next week. How would their local Tesco store respond if they tried this one at the check out? Without being unfair we must bring home to clients that we need money. Be firm and polite. If you give offence just by asking for payment, then the person taking offence has usually got a reason to be defensive. Most people are aware of how the world goes round.

Train your clients so that they expect to pay at each visit, and on collecting animals after surgery. Allowing them to 'pay next time' gets them and you into bad habits. If they decide not to return there is no 'next time'. What if the animal dies between visits? What if the owner dies between visits? What if the owner decides to seek a second opinion? How keen are you going to be to chase up your fees? It may only be a little on each occasion, but it all mounts up.

The main thing to remember is that you are a highly skilled and trained individual. Don't undervalue yourself, or others will do likewise. You work for a fee, and however well you get on with your clients, they still have to pay. If you get complaints about the level of fees, and many people, usually the better-off members of your clientele, can't help having a little dig as they hand over the cash, you can always compare our fees to those of a plumber or a car mechanic, or ask them how many weeks shopping they would get at the supermarket for the spay fee they have just paid, or ask them what they would expect to pay to have their car examined. Another useful ploy is to get hold of the local private hospital's fee structure. The enormous sums charged in the medical sector for similar procedures can emphasise the good value for money that the veterinary profession offers.

Worming

The sad facts are that by far the majority of worming doses are bought from pet shops and the like. Clients either don't think of the practice as a place to get these products, or think that the drugs they buy are as effective as those they would obtain through us. Equally, a large proportion of clients worm their puppies and kittens and then fail to keep up their worming programme once the pet becomes an adult. This is bad for us, bad for the pets and potentially hazardous for the owners.

Client education, communication and training is the key as ever. Fully inform them when they bring their puppies and kittens about worming, not only when the animals are immature, but also when they are adults. Record on their cards when you supply wormers, and ask them if they are up to date with worming when they see you for other complaints. Once you have recorded the treatment, make use of your computer system to send out reminders when the next dose is due. Keep examples of roundworms and tapeworms preserved in little glass pots and have them handy for clients to see and ask about. On newsletters and booster health check reports record the practice advice on worming routines, so that clients are aware that it is necessary to keep up regular worming. Use large posters of worms to grab clients' attention in the waiting room. Make them aware that not only do we provide such treatment, but that it is safe and more effective than the equivalents that they can buy in a pet shop.

Make life a little easier for clients by offering to administer the worming tablets for them. I routinely offer to do this at vaccinations, and in between times the nurses are happy to undertake the task. We make no charge for this, but it is an advantageous arrangement for both clients and practice. Clients do appreciate this service, and it means we don't have to spend time listening to a long list of excuse as to why they are incapable of getting a tablet past the back of Tiddles' tongue.

Flea treatment

Much of the same advice is relevant for flea preparations and treatment. Most preparations are bought from pet shops. The lack of knowledgeable advice, the poor efficacy of the preparations and the sometimes lower safety index of these chemicals means that the client is not doing herself any favours by seeking this option.

Educate clients in the life cycle and persistence of the flea. They will then understand the need for all aspects of treatment, and why we are best placed to supply the correct treatment. Although we know that fleas are the cause of the overwhelming majority of skin problems, clients are not aware of this. They can't always understand that the odd flea that they see from time to time can possibly be responsible for the dramatic skin changes and discomfort their pet is experiencing. Not so long ago it was hard to convince vets that fleas were behind so many of our chronic skins. Many pets simply had prednisolone or 'Ovarid' deficiency.

Stress to clients the importance of 100% per cent flea control, and show how veterinary licensed products are most effective. You can also demonstrate that, although initially more expensive per dose, they are far more cost effective than wasting money on lesser products and spending a fortune on treating the ensuing skin disease.

Skin and ear cases

The problem here is to keep your clients happy while they and their pets endure conditions which are unpleasant, often slow to clear and famously bad at recurring. Once again communication is the key. You must make your clients understand the nature of the disorders, that prolonged treatment is usually necessary and that even the cases which respond well can relapse. If they are aware of the chronic nature of these disorders, they will have realistic expectations of what you are able to do. If you don't win them over, they may eventually decide to try old Mr Easyvet down the road, who will immediately relieve many of the more irritating symptoms with generous doses of steroids, and this will keep the clients happy until their pets develop Cushing's syndrome.

Try to make proper diagnoses of skin and ear cases as early as possible. Use scrapings and swabs at the earliest opportunity. Collect samples of hair to examine and to culture for ringworm. If you suspect atopy, try to perform confirmatory tests, or offer referral to a specialist for intradermal skin testing. All too often we fall into the trap of giving short-term treatment, and repeating on each occasion that the condition recurs. Eventually the client will become frustrated by this. At least if you have a diagnosis to offer, they can comprehend that perhaps the condition won't be cured, or that it might take several months of treatment to clear up.

Discussing treatment options at the outset is important. If you wish to use non-steroid drugs for a skin complaint, you will need to explain that the results will be slower and less dramatic. Clients will usually be quite understanding and patient if they know what to expect, particularly as many have a fear of the dreaded 'steroids'. If, on the other hand, you feel on discussing the case that you have a client who is less interested in a correct scientific approach than a quick cure, you may need to accept that you need to modify your approach and maybe use a dose or two of 'Itchyfix'.

One bad habit which owners have is to hold on to drugs once they feel that a complaint has cleared up. Some clients have drug cupboards at home which rival our own. Not only does this indicate that the patient hasn't received its full course of treatment, but it also means that by the time Scabbers is presented to you it has already had a selection of drugs tried on it, some dating back to the dark ages. This may make your task difficult. For one thing, the only bugs left are likely to be multiple resistant super-cyberbugs, and for another every time you offer a bottle of medicine the owner will dismiss it with a 'tried that'. Feel free to communicate to your clients the full range of reasons which make the retaining of drugs a bad idea. Explain that they are inducing resistant bacteria, limiting the range of drugs which will be effective for their pet. Tell them that by using old medications they are not only using ineffective preparations, but may be introducing further infective organisms to their poor pet's eyes or ears. Point out the instructions on the drug boxes or your drug labels which tell them to discard unused medicine 7 or 14 or 30 days after opening. Stress that the expiry date on a bottle of drops only refers to the unopened, fresh product.

Skin diseases can be the most rewarding and interesting of cases to deal with. Dermatology is really not a hard subject, as can be seen by the rash of certificates in dermatology which abound. It simply involves a logical approach, and patience on the part of the paying customer. Talk to your clients, and you will be allowed all the time you need.

Neutering

You may encounter some resistance to neutering on the part of your clients. (I am of course referring to neutering of their pets here.) This is particularly noticeable in the case of male dogs, and not all the resistance is offered by male owners, although they often do react to the mention of castration by instinctively covering up their own assets. So important to a man's ego are the contents of his dog's scrotum, that in the States it is possible to buy artificial testicles, called 'Neuticles'. These were apparently developed to 'prevent psychological trauma in neutered dogs', but it is fairly obvious whose psyche we are really dealing with.

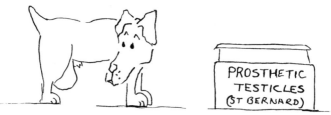

Firstly you need to decide whether you are in favour of blanket neutering or a more selective approach. Be aware of the advantages and possible drawbacks in each species. Once you know where you stand, you are in a position to convince owners of the rights and wrongs of the process. I have seen some comments by one or two vets that neutering (of canines) is an unnecessary mutilation, an unnatural process carried out simply for our convenience. Is this so? Would the same people advocate leaving cats entire, so that queens would soon be worn out from overproduction of kittens, toms would be un-homeable and FIV rampant and there would be basketfuls of kittens flushed down toilets or sent in black bags to the tip? The keeping of pets is unnatural and we already mould cats and dogs to the shape and character that we desire. Isn't it kinder to them to remove the frustrations of an unfulfilled desire to breed? What about the undoubted health benefits which neutering can provide? The reduction in cases of malignant mammary tumours, avoidance of pyometra and reproductive tract neoplasia, prevention of prostatic disease and perianal adenomas. To be sure we must balance any benefits against the possible ill effects of neutering: incontinence, weight gain and coat changes.

It is for you, who are in a position to understand the full implications of neutering, to decide upon your stance, and then you may communicate your opinion to your clients. Your advice will be listened to, if not always acted upon. Many of the clients' fears about neutering are irrational, not based upon science. For instance, why do clients who think nothing of having a bitch spayed, baulk at castration of their dogs? Castration is such a minor procedure in comparison to ovariohysterectomy. Bitches lose just as many hormones as dogs do when neutered, so why the concerns about 'changing his character' when they don't seem to worry about her character? As far as control of unwanted births goes, bitches may have two litters a year, with maybe six puppies in each. A fit dog might mate a bitch a day if the fancy took him, and be responsible for hundreds of litters in a year. Talk facts, and talk them early on. Start to discuss this when young puppies and kittens are brought in, so that clients have plenty of time to discuss their own wishes and ask you any questions. Once clients are able to make informed decisions, you are likely to have a steady supply of candidates to practice your neutering technique upon.

Alternative therapy

There is an increasing mistrust of modern medicines amongst the general public, whether for themselves or for their pets. Unfortunately, most alternative medicines or therapies are not subject to the rigid controls which our scientific remedies must undergo. Clients also don't seem to expect so much of them, so that they may purchase several courses of treatment which appear to give little benefit to the pet, and yet the owner is quite happy. If we start a course of treatment, sometimes owners will phone when they arrive home from the surgery, complaining that their pet hasn't been cured yet. Remember also that many complaints will improve spontaneously, regardless of whether they receive treatment from us, the medicine man down the road or Mystic Meg.

You do need to be open-minded in your approach, or you may upset and lose clients. They are entitled to their beliefs, although they are often based upon flawed arguments and incorrect data or interpretation. If you simply dismiss alternative medicines as homeopathetic your client may see you as too dogmatic and narrow minded. If asked for my position on alternative remedies, I usually state that I am open-minded, but that I need scientific proof rather than hearsay before I could possibly recommend such therapy. On the other hand, if clients wish to try it, and it doesn't interfere with the treatment regime I am using, then at least alternative medicines don't usually do any harm. That is not always the case, however, and you need to be aware of the active agents in herbal medicines in case the owner is unwittingly doing their pet some ill.

If dealing with a client who prefers not to use drugs such as antibiotics and steroids unless absolutely necessary, you may find the experience somewhat uplifting. We are often placed in the position of having to provide drugs for a quick fix to keep clients happy and justify our fees. Many cases can be treated quite successfully without resorting to the big guns, and it is rewarding to work with a client who will use dietary therapy, patience and preparations such as probiotics.

Working on the principle that if you can't beat them you may as well join them, work with local practitioners of therapies such as osteopathy and acupuncture so that if you are faced with a client who is going to seek such treatment, you can refer them to a friendly face who will work with you rather than against you.

Encouraging well-behaved pets

Love is blind, and many owners of unruly or unpleasant dogs are oblivious to their failings. You can improve your relations with these pets and do a favour to most people and dogs that they are going to meet by encouraging good behaviour. Many dogs which we see with personality disorders as adults have suffered from bad experiences or insufficient experiences during their crucial formative period of up to 16 weeks of age. Ensure that you make owners of new puppies aware that they only have really quite a small window of opportunity to allow good socialisation and habituation. Give plenty of advice and guidance as to what owners should be doing with puppies in these formative weeks. Encourage them to take advantage of puppy classes, and then training classes.

If you have an interest in behavioural therapy, encourage owners of disturbed pets to seek your help. If it isn't your forte, either have someone in the practice that you can recommend or a local behavioural therapist that you are familiar and happy with. Many clients put up with much inconvenience simply because they are unaware that anything can be done to improve their pet's behaviour. At the same time the pets are experiencing high levels of stress and are not really having a happy and fulfilled life. So don't grit your teeth when Zebedee bounces all over you or chews up your stethoscope. Ask the owner if he has noticed anything abnormal about the dog's behaviour and let him know that help is available.

- Persuasion of clients is important for pets' health, professional satisfaction and practice turnover
- Clients can't be relied upon to know what is best for their pets
- Vets have a natural reluctance to sell services, which needs to be overcome
- Persuade, don't bully
- Personal experience is a good tool for persuasion – use the 'my pet' or 'my friend' approach
- It isn't up to the vet to save or spend their clients' money
- Advice which is paid for is perceived to be more valuable than free advice
- It is better to advise laboratory tests, investigative procedures and clinical diets at an early point
- Be open about the fact that treatment costs money, and provide clients with a guide to the costs early on

6

How to look good

How not to look bad?

Monday afternoon, you're ten minutes late to see the first appointment. As you slouch into the consulting room a glimpse of Day-Glo sock peeks from between your frayed jeans leg and your well-worn trainers. A lank lock of hair falls over one eye. As you smear it back onto your head, you recall that when it came to a choice between your fifth pint or going home for a bath and a shampoo, you chose beer. Perhaps the reheated *balti* you had for lunch wasn't such a good idea. Apart from the interesting effects it is producing as it greets the remains of last night's bitter, the receptionist did seem to recoil rather as she passed you the afternoon's record cards. You have forgotten to bring a new white coat in as well, and there are distinct stains from the morning's encounter with Mrs Dainty's Cavalier's anal glands. Well, less like stains, really, more sort of scratch and sniff patches. Still, if you lean up against the sink with your right side they are not too obvious.

Better get started. Looking at the name on the card, you call 'Mrs Cameron' into the waiting room. No client appears, so you move to the consulting room door while trying a hearty sort of call: 'MRS CAMERON!'. Of the three men seated in the waiting room, the largest, a docker from the local port, slowly unfolds himself from his seat.

'Ah! Good afternoon Mr Cameron. Come in. This must be Squidgy.'

'This is Fluffy. Squidgy was hit by a car last Thursday and you put her to sleep.'

'Oh.'

Fluffy has a couple of troubles today. She has been rubbing her bottom along the ground, and has also developed quite a harsh cough. You tackle the bottom first. Asking Mr Cameron to hold her upright, you advance upon her with your gloved finger forward. Something, however, seems to be wrong.

'That's funny. I can't feel anything at all in her glands.'

'Do they grow back then?' inquires the client.

'Eh?'

'You removed her anal glands last year.'

'Oh.'

Thankfully, a quick comb through Fluffy's fur reveals a clutch of fleas. After informing the client that he'll have to get some effective flea treatment ('But I bought the drops from you not six weeks ago!'), you turn your attention to the cough. You place the stethoscope gently against the chest.

'Whoah!' you cry, stepping back a pace, 'That's a heck of a heart murmur. Your dog has congestive heart failure leading to her cough.'

'Don't the pills she's been having keep that under control?'

'Eh?'

'You've been giving her medication for her heart for two years now and it's working very well. I don't know if it's of any importance, but she was in kennels for a week. Came out seven days ago.'

'Oh.'

As you commence treatment for Fluffy's kennel cough, you explain that you are injecting an anti-inflammatory to make her throat more comfortable.

'Will that be Ok with her Antistiff medicine?'

'Eh?'

'You started her on the Antistiff last year for her arthritic hip. It's very good. Isn't that an anti-inflammatory?'

'Oh.'

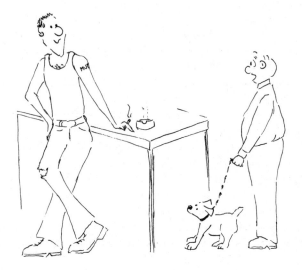

Things haven't been going smoothly, made worse by Fluffy's loud squealing as you caught a tender spot with the injection you administered. Better soften Mr Cameron up a bit.

'Good win for the Blues last night wasn't it?'

'I support the Reds. Have done man and boy. That's why I'm wearing a Reds shirt.'

'Oh.'

Time to call a halt to this session, enjoyable as you are finding it. You escort Mr Cameron to the reception desk where no one is to be seen. A gentle call produces no staff, so you have to go in search of your receptionist. Reassuring Mr Cameron that she'll be along in a minute, you carefully call in your next client. A few minutes later there is a knock on the door. The receptionist puts her head round the corner.

'Excuse me, but did you mean to prescribe Sindypox tablets for Fluffy? You know she's got a penicillin allergy?'

'Oh.'

Not a great demonstration of the art of client management, but these are all examples of what can happen if there is no attention to detail, no pride in one's work. The art of looking good is more an exercise in avoiding looking bad. In this chapter we will cover some of the areas where you can make a good impression and how to do it.

Be older

Sadly there is one way of looking good to clients which may be beyond you at present. There is no doubt that many clients regard older members of the profession with more respect. Part of the reason for this is that over the years these senior vets have learned how to look after their clients and what they like. The purpose of this book is after all to give you a slight head start in making you aware of the range of non-clinical details that you need to cover in practice. Partly, though, there is simply an assumption that more years under the belt means more experience and so older vets command more respect. This can be frustrating for the young vet who knows that she is just as capable as her older colleague and far more up to date in veterinary science, and who sees minor slips and lapses by an older colleague either ignored or forgiven by clients when they would probably pass comment had she been in error. Don't worry. If you perform your work efficiently and are pleasant to clients and compassionate to your patients you will soon be regarded with respect and affection by those same clients. The day when a client asks for you in preference to one of the more experienced members of the practice is a red letter day, and it won't be long in coming.

The role of lay staff

Preparation is everything when you are getting ready to meet your public, and your lay staff can prime you nicely. They can indicate to you whether Mr or Mrs or Miss has come today, which animal they have brought and any snippets of information they have been passed. This puts you in a good position to discuss the client's holiday or their daughter's wedding.

Lay staff should also talk you up, not to the detriment of other vets in the practice, but so that you are given a good image in the public's view. They should show confidence in your ability and point out your strong points without inferring that you have weak points. They should cover up for you if you have forgotten to do something or made a slight error, such as prescribing the wrong strength tablets or forgotten to phone a client at the time you had promised. In short they should act as a PR machine for the vets in the clinic because everyone benefits if the vets have a good image.

Communication – vet to vet and vet to staff

Communication is vital if you, your colleagues and your lay staff are to look their best. This involves talking to each other. Sometimes it can appear as though each piece of information gleaned by members of a practice is treated like a state secret. Facts and laboratory results, responses to treatment, complaints, praise, progress reports – all have to be prised from each other. Talk to each other. Appear interested when you are being told something. It can be frustrating and discouraging for lay staff to pass on information to a vet who gives every impression of either not caring or being too busy to listen. Discuss cases amongst yourselves, as well as your approach to various diseases. Only in this way will the practice develop a consistent mode of action. It does not inspire confidence when an owner finds two vets in the same practice working up similar problems in completely different manners.

Similarly, take the time to record information thoroughly on your records. The transition from paper records to computer screens has not encouraged this. There is a tendency to write less and less, until sometimes only the bare facts of what treatment has been administered are recorded.

This causes difficulties both when notes are passed to another practice, and when other members of the practice come to deal with the case. When writing notes, assume that the client may not be seeing you the next time, and record any relevant information about the case, including your differential list and your planned course of action. If, for instance, you were treating a case of otitis externa, and you were on the point of performing a bacterial swab or an examination under anaesthetic should there be no improvement over the ensuing five days, record this. Otherwise, if you are ill or unavailable the next time the client brings his dog, your colleague may either carry on the fruitless course of treatment, or else dive in with his own investigations, thereby both undermining your reputation, and perhaps heading down a different diagnostic route to the one you had chosen.

If you are going on holiday, update your fellow vets on all your ongoing cases, including those you weren't expecting to see. It is frustrating to lose control of a case because a colleague has taken it on in your absence, yet they may have no option if they don't know your mind. Keep lay staff informed of cases where the owners may contact the surgery for advice, enabling the staff to handle routine enquiries about the case. You may also inform staff or agencies taking the phones at night or at the weekend of cases which are ongoing and may require delicate handling or extra reassurance. It is dispiriting for a client who has been bringing her dog in every day during the week to find that the night staff have no idea who she is. Remember that clients like to feel as though they are the most important clients at the practice, and they find it flattering if their pet is readily recognised.

Communication – vet to client

If there is one point which should be gleaned from this book as a whole, it is that communicating with your clients, educating them, discussing cases with them and explaining their pets' problems and your line of treatment is all of prime importance. Keep in touch with your clients and they are far less likely to be disgruntled or confused by your actions. Surely the commonest reason for clients seeking a second opinion is misunderstanding between the client and the vet or practice. The client may not realise the extent of the investigations being performed, or the nature of the treatment being given or the chronic nature of the disease or the high regard that she is held in at the practice, all because she was never told any of this. Many a time I have done a little résumé of the condition for a client seeking a second opinion with me, and she has looked at me as though she had never heard any of this before. The original vet was no doubt extremely competent, but the client had no way of knowing because he never took the time to talk to her.

You need to tailor the amount and complexity of information that you give a client for each case. Some clients are not as capable of absorbing technical details, nor do they want to worry about them. All clients, however, want to be told something about what is wrong with their pet. Follow up what you tell interested clients with a handout if the case is complicated. Conditions such as diabetes, Cushing's syndrome, OCD or atopy are hard for clients to grasp. Help them by providing them with the information that allows them to develop some background knowledge. If the handouts are produced by the practice, it allows your views on how to diagnose and manage the condition to be expressed.

Take the time to keep on communicating with clients as a case progresses. Don't necessarily wait for them to come to the next consultation. Telephone them to see if they are coping with the tablets, whether there are any side effects and whether you have managed to bring about an improvement. Let the clients know that they are important to you, and they will respond with their loyalty.

Keeping to appointment times

Mrs Hargreave was a new client. On her first visit to the clinic, she booked an appointment to have her cat's booster vaccination. The appointed time came and went, and she duly arrived 25 minutes late. She was most taken aback to receive a very mild rebuke from the receptionist, who thought that perhaps she had lost her way having not been to us before. Oh no, she replied, it was her standard practice when visiting her doctor's surgery to arrive 20 or so minutes late for her appointment, because she then didn't have to wait too long before he was ready to see her.

Clients may be accustomed to being kept waiting long past their allotted appointment times by other service providers, but that doesn't mean to say that they are happy with the situation. On the contrary it is a constant source of irritation, and may actually put them off visiting those providers, whether they be the doctor, the vet or the local planning officer, unless they really need to go. We don't want to discourage our clients from visiting the practice, nor do we wish to give them cause for complaint. Make every effort to keep as close as possible to your appointment times. We all appreciate that it is difficult for us to predict how long each client will take. Not only is the nature of the problem unknown, but the time taken may depend upon the level of co-operation from both client and pet. On top of this, clients who may grumble because they are seen late then proceed to hold court, ensuring that not only do they receive their full allocation of time, but they eat well into the next client's appointment as well. We can improve the situation. When appointments are booked, ask the reception staff to enquire about the reason for the appointment, how many animals are coming and if there are likely to be any complications. If they recognise a client who habitually outstays their welcome, they might book a double appointment for them. Feel free to charge extra – your time is what you have to sell. Be polite but firm with clients if they are taking up too much time. On quiet days it is good to chat to them, but not when you are behind with appointments. Make use of your lay staff if you are running late. Once you have decided on the treatment required, they are quite capable of administering it and giving routine advice.

Clients do appreciate appointments running close to time. Everyone is busy these days, and we need to make a trip to the vet convenient as well as enjoyable. If the client is stressed because he has had to wait and he has something else to do or somewhere to go once he has finished with us, it isn't going to help our relationship with him. On the other hand, if your appointments usually run smoothly and to time, clients will tell their friends and you will further enhance your practice's reputation.

Promising to contact clients

When taking blood samples, skin scrapings or the like, or if you are looking up some research into a pet's condition, clients very much appreciate being called with results or a progress report. Far better that you are first to contact them, rather than waiting for the client to call chasing the results. Similarly, when their pets are in for radiography or ultrasound examination, or other investigations, they are grateful to hear from you at the earliest opportunity, rather than having to worry all day until they collect their animal.

It is important if you have promised to contact the client that you try to keep to your promise. I usually record on the card the date and time that I called, so that if there is no reply I can at least show that I have tried. If there is an answer machine use it, but not to leave important results on. Explain why you are calling and ask the client to call back at their convenience. Have a fallback, so that you ask the client to call you at a certain time if they haven't heard from you first, but try to beat them to it. If you are busy, and the results or information can be passed on by lay staff, make use of your nurses and reception staff. Be warned that once you have promised to contact the client, they will remember and hold it against you if you fail.

Be confident

Do you remember the one about the worried worker who went to see the company doctor? 'Doc, I'm haven't been feeling too good lately. Can you help me?' says the worker. 'Have you been feeling tired and listless?' asked the doctor. 'Yes' came the reply. 'Been experiencing trouble passing water, lost your appetite and developed a purple rash around your neck?' 'Yes, yes! Those are my symptoms exactly! What's the matter with me Doc?' 'Beats me' replies the medical man, 'I've had those symptoms for weeks and I've got no idea.'

You should have a confident and reassuring air when dealing with clients. They are paying you to know what to do when their pets are ill. They are not likely to be impressed if you stare at their pet in consternation, shaking your head, and asking them if they have any idea what is likely to be wrong. No one expects you to know everything, but you should know what to do to find out what the problem is. There is no shame in admitting that you cannot make a diagnosis straight away. In fact I would venture that it is a rash man who announces definitely that he knows exactly what is wrong with a sick pet. You should be able to offer a differential list however, and have an action plan to either investigate and allow identification of the disorder, or to try logical treatment. You may well be panicking under your calm exterior, thinking that this looks like nothing you've ever experienced, but you have colleagues to discuss a case with and plenty of backup behind the scenes. As long as the clients know that you are not completely stumped, they will trust you.

Clients are usually reassured if you can offer a diagnosis, whether straight away or after a few preliminary investigations. I would caution against being too definite, but I would also advise that you do offer them a diagnosis, however tentative. Animals are funny things, and they do have a habit of trying to conceal the true nature of their illness from you, so always leave yourself an escape route, allowing you to modify your diagnosis without appearing to do a complete volte-face.

Keeping up to date with current therapies

Veterinary science is changing at a great pace. Our knowledge of disease mechanisms and aetiologies is increasing daily. New ideas on treatment appear with frightening regularity, and truths which we held dear a few years ago are being challenged and overturned all the time. Perhaps the present time is seeing the fastest change in medical and veterinary science ever – and that statement may be true even if you read this book half a century after the time of writing. You may have sighed a huge sigh of relief on graduation, fondly imagining that your days of study and research are over, that you were then fully equipped for life in the workplace. Sadly you will find that you need to keep fully abreast of all current developments if you are to remain in the front line of veterinary medicine. This is not all bad news, as new ideas are stimulating, and you are now in a position to not only read or hear about these new ideas, but to evaluate them in the field and add your own valuable voice to those of other reviewers.

Your clients are also becoming more and more knowledgeable. They have been given a useful insight into the veterinary world through the numerous television shows which present all the common illnesses and a good smattering of more exotic ones as well. Even more frightening are the 'internet clients' who, once given the name of a disorder, spend the wee hours of the morning trawling the world wide web looking at obscure web sites which purport to tell them all they ever wanted to know about hepatic lipidopathy or Helicobacter infection in gerbils. The beauty and the difficulty of the internet is that there is no censorship or approval necessary. Anyone with an idea or a theory is free to publish it for all to see. Many of your clients will subscribe to the view that if something is in print, it must be true. This is inaccurate enough when dealing with the somewhat dubious reports that find their way into the tabloid press. Unfortunately some clients are unable to make the distinction, and you will from time to time be presented with some exotic ideas disseminated via the web. It seems that the more loony the author, the more persuasive the web content. The only way to retain your client's faith in the face of such information is to show them that you are keeping up to date with developments in the field. Let them know that you attend continuing education, and that you read journals. Don't necessarily dismiss 'internet advice' out of hand. Offer to look at it and give the client an informed opinion on the content. Deal similarly with snippets of information which clients pick up from television, papers and magazines.

Keeping up to date with current affairs

Your clients will not only expect you to be fully up to date with clinical developments, but also to be conversant with current veterinary affairs. You are the interface for them between what is reported in the media and the man in the street. Recent topics which clients might have wanted to discuss include the BSE crisis, the changing of the quarantine laws and various health scares. You need to be able to provide facts, correct misconceptions and have an opinion. By doing this you can both provide a service to your clients and show them that you are keeping abreast of current issues.

Know your breeds

Pity the poor vet. Clients regularly comment on how much easier it must be to be a doctor than a vet, because they only have to learn about one species. They little know the extent of our problem. Imagine being a doctor, but in the year 2299, when Earth is the equivalent of a Plastic Coffee service station just off the intergalactic highway, the I G 25. You not only have to know and understand human physiology, but the biology and medical complaints of innumerable alien species which pass through. Many of them are quite similar to the species you learnt about at medical school, but some are truly strange. Many you can't even recognise. Some are carnivorous, some are obligate vegetarians. Some can fly. Many have a respiratory apparatus quite different to our own. They may have no diaphragm, and pump air back and forth across a gas exchange unit by means of bellows. Others absorb oxygen through a liquid medium. Many have highly modified limbs, while others have no limbs at all. Some are homeothermic, others are poikilothermic. A few speak some words of human languages, but give no indication that they understand what they are saying, which can give rise to amusing scenarios when they pipe up in inappropriate situations.

Well friends and colleagues, welcome to our working world. The field of medical care is roughly broken into two. Doctors take care of one species, veterinarians look after the rest. Unfortunately, we are quite likely to be presented with hundreds of different species to care for, even in a fairly tame small animal practice. Even the most critical client can't expect you to be familiar with every exotic species and breed, but we should be familiar with as many as possible, not only to impress clients, but so that we have a basic idea of their peculiarities and requirements.

Start with dog and cat breeds. Have a working knowledge of the common breeds, and for dogs, of what their purpose is. Each locality will have a population of breeds more common in that area, in addition to the normal retrievers, German Shepherds and Westies. Local people like you to recognise their pet breeds, and to tell them what a fine specimen theirs is. You will have local breeders of cats and dogs increasing the numbers of their specialist breeds locally. In most cases it doesn't matter if you can't tell a Samoyed from a Munsterlander, or a British Blue from a Russian Blue, but you are supposed to be knowledgeable about animals. Owners have a little more faith in you if you can recognise their dog. You will often hear them ask if you are used to treating Lancashire Heelers or Bouviers de Flandres. Many less common breeds, because of their small gene pool, also have congenital or hereditary disorders which are disproportionally represented in those breeds and this knowledge may prove useful to you.

Rabbits and guinea pigs are becoming ever more popular pets for those clients with a busy lifestyle. They are not all just 'rabbit' or 'guinea pig', at least to their owners. There are breeds and types, and clients will be delighted if you recognise their Flemish Giant or American Crested.

Parrot owners are a singular breed in themselves. They are loathe to believe that the ordinary vet in the street is capable of ministering to their pets, and this is a suspicion reinforced if the vet cannot identify the species of bird she is examining, cannot tell the difference between a male and female budgie or cockatiel or is unaware of the diet of the particular parrot that is ill.

More exotic species abound. If I am honest, you will usually need to be told the species of reptile which is brought to you. There are many similar types of reptiles and often they haven't been properly identified by the dealer or pet shop owner. There are a few species which are easier to keep and therefore more common, so you should be familiar with Herman's and Spur-thighed tortoises, green iguanas and bearded dragons, garter snakes and king snakes.

Have a selection of books on dog, cat and small mammal breeds, parrot species and reptiles available. When dealing with exotics you may find that a good book on the biology and natural history of the animal is more useful than a veterinary book, since you can use it to check the environment and diet of the patient.

Dress code

Sorry to bring this up again, but if you want to be taken seriously, you need to look the part. Not all your clients will be regulars who have had time to adjust to your eccentricities, your hippie jeans, your flashing-light trainers, your revolving bow tie. All very jolly and making a statement that you are not one of the crowd. Ask yourself this, though. If your child was ill and you took her to the doctors, would you want to see a medic who looked the part or an extra from Barnum? Amongst your clients will be owners who have been up all night with their vomiting puppy, pensioners investing their week's allowance on their consultation with you and children bringing their family pet for euthanasia. They deserve to be attended to by someone who looks as though he is dealing with their problems soberly. No need to go over the top, but be presentable and don't give offence, however unwittingly.

Professional attitude

What constitutes having a professional attitude? Hard to define, but it encapsulates courtesy to clients and colleagues (both in your practice and outside of it), a fair and even-handed approach, honesty with your clients, respect for your clients whatever their status (financial, social, mental or otherwise), diligence, discretion and the endeavour to keep your knowledge and skills up to date. Achieve this and you will be respected in your own right by your clients, staff and peers.

It is relatively easy for us to attain these standards when in our working environment, but we live in the community in which we work. Inevitably we come into contact with clients of the practice daily during our 'private' lives. We must attempt to maintain a reasonably professional attitude in our life outside the practice, because although we can easily make the distinction between our working and off-duty personas, our clients may not find it so easy. If they see you rather the worse for wear in the local pub on a Saturday night, or involved in a brawl at the Sunday League soccer match, or shouting at the check-out girl in the supermarket, their opinion of you as a vet will be affected. Nobody said it was fair, but it is life. You wouldn't expect to see a nun rolling down the street with a bottle of gin swinging from one hand and a slim panatela in the other, or involved in a slanging match with a rabbi from the community synagogue, even if it was outside the convent. We may not wear a physical uniform outside the practice, but we are labelled all the same.

Be sure that you don't discuss clients' affairs or cases in public, and certainly don't name names. Before you honk your horn at that incompetent driver blocking your passage or lean out of the window to remonstrate with him, be sure that he isn't one of the practice's valuable clients. Don't air your views on the utter foolishness of people who own Egyptian huskies in case the secretary of the local breed society is in earshot. Don't make pronouncements or voice opinions which may be too controversial or contradict practice policy or official veterinary wisdom. Never criticise other vets in public. Basically, think before you speak or act. It isn't really that hard. Get into the habit and it will come naturally.

A sympathetic approach

However clever, annoying, supercilious, silly, irritating, aggressive, pleasant, unhelpful, adoring, suspicious or otherwise engaging your clients may be, they have brought their animals to you because they care about them to some degree. Remember that many of the less endearing traits displayed by owners are brought about by their worries and concerns about the well-being of their pets. Whatever your personal feelings about a client, you must present a sympathetic front in your dealing with both human and animal.

There may be times when a client has quite clearly caused or exacerbated a pet's condition by their ignorance or neglect. This doesn't automatically mean that they don't have the pet's best interests at heart. Think of all those obese cats and dogs you see daily, their state of fatness brought on purely by their owners' overindulgence. You can be strict and lay down the law with those owners, but you must not give them to think that you hold them guilty of wilful cruelty. Owners don't want to be told that they are unkind to animals, and there are plenty of vets who won't point this out to them to choose from.

There are times when it may seem difficult to provide sympathy to clients. The first appointment of the evening, which turns out to be a euthanasia, but the owners want to go through a lengthy process of persuasion, while you are hopelessly thinking of your mounting list of waiting clients. The client who calls in the middle of morning operations to talk about her ailing cat which you have in the hospital, while your nurse keeps significantly appearing in front of you, indicating that she would like to be finished in time for lunch. The client who insists on phoning you after every puppy is born, between the hours of 2 and 5 a.m. It may take the patience of a saint, but if you are able to present a calm and reassuring front to these clients, whatever you privately feel, your reputation will suffer no harm. You will develop methods for the polite hurrying up of people. Be sure that they don't give offence or lead your clients to suspect that they are less important than another client.

Whenever possible, provide plenty of sympathy to your patients. It is usually evident to an owner whether a vet genuinely likes animals or not. They are willing to forgive many minor hiccups and indiscretions if the vet has a good rapport with the pets. I do know vets who have the bedside manner of an Alf Garnett, but who are held in high regard by their clients because of their clear affinity with the dogs and cats brought to them. It usually comes naturally to us to treat animals with care and compassion. Just remember to be as caring to pets that you find physically repulsive, vile charactered, or which have personality deficiencies.

Surgery

Some of us take naturally to surgery; others will struggle to achieve full confidence. One thing is for sure: clients are by and large completely oblivious to what goes on under the surface of their pets. What they care about is the number of stitches, how the wound looks and how much hair you have clipped off. Consequently, if you want to look like a good surgeon, I would advise taking a little time to ensure that your skin closure is tidy, that the clipping is neat and level and that there is as little mess as possible on your patient when it is collected. I have seen examples of surgery on humans where a high-powered consultant surgeon has performed miracles of surgery inside a patient, then left a junior doctor to practice his suturing skills on the skin wound. The patient has then looked as though the local play group have had a go at doctors and nurses.

Small neat wounds are impressive to clients and are usually less uncomfortable for patients, leading to a faster recovery and less chance of wound interference. Be careful, though, that you don't get too carried away. An acquaintance was very proud of his bitch spay wounds, which used to be quite tiny. One day he surpassed himself and managed to spay a young Labrador bitch through a wound which he closed with one small horizontal mattress suture. Bursting with pride, he couldn't wait to discharge the bitch that afternoon. The appointed hour arrived and he presented the client with his Labrador, finishing his post-operative advice with a flourish as he demonstrated the tiny incision. The client, unfortunately, was less than impressed: 'You mean to say you've charged me all this money for that tiny wound?' The vet concerned now contents himself with more normal-sized incisions.

However skilfully and carefully surgery is performed, there are many complications waiting to happen. Thankfully most of these are minor and easily dealt with. Some can be quite major, involving more work to correct than the original procedure. Our policy with complications arising from routine surgical procedures is not to charge clients for putting things right. Even if the problem has arisen because of the patient's awkwardness or the client's negligence, we will still undertake to correct the problem. This has the advantage of forestalling any queries about cost that the client may put forward, spare us the agonies of deciding whether a problem has come about because of something we have done insufficiently well or whether it is a complication beyond our control, and it pleases clients. If you adopt this policy, and believe me clients appreciate it, be sure that you don't make this an admission that the complication is your fault. Your professional indemnity insurers would not be impressed with that. Rather say that the complication is something that may well happen, but that as a practice policy you normally will take care of complications as a gesture of goodwill. The exceptions for us are the operation where complications are to be expected, where the client has insisted upon a procedure, perhaps against our better judgement, or where the client really has been wilfully or repeatedly negligent.

Contact owners after operations

Clients are worried when they leave their treasured pets with us for surgery. We take it all in our stride, and often the patients do as well. The clients are the ones whose imaginations run riot, and who expect the worst at every opportunity. It will go a long way towards setting their minds at rest if they are kept up to date with proceedings. When a surgical procedure has been completed, however simple, get your nurse to call the client to let them know how things have gone. Once the patient has made a good recovery, arrange for another telephone call to let the client know. This simple courtesy is much appreciated, and needn't take up any of your time at all.

Progress reports on in-patients

Once again, clients worry about their pets when they have to spend time at the practice. They are concerned about the progress of the condition, how their pets are coping without their owners, whether they are eating and going to the toilet properly, whether they are playing with the toys that they have been left with. Rather than leaving your clients to fret, arrange for them to have regular updates from the nurse in charge of kennels or in-patients. A couple of calls a day are not too onerous. If the clients are out when called, leave a message on their answering machine. Don't obstruct a client's access to their pet any more than is necessary. Some in-patients are terminal cases. Some may die at unexpected times, or decline rapidly. Don't deprive owners of the chance to see and talk to their pets just because they are hospitalised. Be sure that all in-patients are kept in clean and comfortable conditions. Visitors will inevitably look at other pets apart from their own when they come, so it is not sufficient just to spruce up their pet's kennel when you expect them.

Above all, do your best not to make an owner find out that their pet has died when they are calling you. It is inevitable that some in-patients will not make it – they are hospitalised because they are seriously ill, but when one does die you must make every effort to inform the owner first. This is not a task for the lay staff. The client must hear this from you. You will need to reassure them that the pet was receiving the best of care, and that it wasn't suffering. There is a case for a small white lie if the pet had an uncomfortable end. It serves no purpose to give the client all the gory details.

Follow-up calls

Out of sight, out of mind, they say. Your clients will be impressed if you can show them that this is not the case where their pets are concerned. After surgical procedures, or after hospitalised patients have returned home, schedule a telephone call the following day and thereafter as appropriate to check on their progress. You may also like to check on other cases that you have seen and started on treatment. You or your lay staff can do this. It is not only reassuring for the client, but also useful for you. You can note the progress on the pet's records, answer any queries the client will have, discuss any side effects or developments in the disease and ensure that they are giving the medication at the right dose, the right frequency and by the correct route. Don't make the call a substitute for a consultation, but show that you care.

Noting details on the records

You can spare yourself much time and embarrassment, as well as appearing even more efficient than you undoubtedly are, by making good use of notes on patients' record cards or computer records. The following are some useful items that you or your lay staff should be sure to record.

Entire or neutered, with age of neutering if mature when done
Heart murmur, with date detected, most recent grade and character
Missing organs or limbs. e.g. anal sacs, spleen, kidney, and I'm not joking about the limbs
Diagnosed allergies
Sensitivities to drugs
Aversion to injections, including specific examples of drugs or routes to avoid
Aggression rating, including sensitive body areas
Effective sedative doses
Insurance status
Hereditary diseases in the pet's relatives
Liking for treats at the surgery

No doubt you can add extensively to the list. Once these notes are made, take the time to read them. It is embarrassing to inject a dog with cephalexin, and only then to read that it has a habit of erupting with crusting pustular dermatitis whenever it so much as sniffs the drug. Clients are notoriously slow at warning you about their dog's aversion to being handled. Many is the time I have had a dog's mouth open and peered down its throat while the owner looked on with a beatific smile. Only as I close the mouth and stand back do they pipe up: 'Well! He's never let anyone do that before.' Spare your colleagues damage to their extremities by passing on such little titbits of information.

Noting personal details on records

As well as being aware of a patient's clinical peculiarities, it makes a good impression if you can be aware of some of the pets' and owners' personal details. This isn't strictly relevant to the examination, but it flatters the owner and also helps you to make pertinent conversation. Some examples of possible topics for inclusion follow.

Birthdays, pets and owners
Preferences, such as type of medication (tablets, powders, liquids), feeding, male or female vets
Ability to administer medication
Prizes or awards won, by pet or owner
Personal landmarks, e.g. weddings, children's wedding, birth of children, death of husband/wife
Favourite football team
Where the client went on holiday
Concerns about certain medicines/vaccines
Liking for alternative medicines/therapies
Where the pet came from, e.g. dog's home, one of your breeders, via your practice
Previous bad experiences, so as to avoid repeating them

A moment or two taken to record the details can greatly increase your stock with your clientele. Even if they are aware that you don't have an encyclopaedic memory and are using cribs to help you, the fact that you take the trouble is appreciated. If you are putting this on a computer, you may need to register with the Data Protection Agency.

Being prepared

Take a moment or two before calling in the client to familiarise yourself with the case, especially if it isn't one you have been dealing with. One of the most common complaints from clients is that they 'never see the same vet twice' and have to recite the whole history of the case over and over again. Good recording of case histories and a vet's thinking on the case will standardise the practice's approach to a case, making life much easier when a colleague has to see a patient and relieving much of the irritation caused to clients. Be sure that you can talk to the client knowledgeably about the case, fully aware of the treatment so far, investigations performed and response to therapy.

You should be able to make an educated guess from the card as to which pet a client is bringing in, enabling you to greet the pet by name. If your reception staff haven't provided a clue as to whether Mr, Mrs or Miss X has brought the pet, identifying the patient in the waiting room should allow you to politely call in the client. Try to avoid the rather abrupt and impersonal summoning of clients by surnames alone.

Coping with badly behaved pets

You may think differently, but to dear old Mrs Sweetness, Ripper the Rottweiler, Genghis the cat or Atilla the Bun are her little darlings. They may behave appallingly through out-and-out aggression, nervousness or terror. Whatever the reason, you will gain points if you can deal with them calmly, without undue force, harsh words and large iron bars. I would never advocate that veterinary staff or clients should be put at risk. I also agree that bad behaviour in pets should be corrected where possible. However, I don't really think that the stressful environment of a consulting room is really the place to achieve very effective corrective behavioural therapy. What will work wonders is a calm approach, confidence, sympathy, bribery and a sense of how far to push things before provoking an attack or a severe fear reaction. I am firmly of the opinion that many pets' reluctance to tamely receive our tender ministrations is a consequence of past bad experiences at the hands of veterinary staff. This may have been rough handling and poor injection technique when young or forcible examination of painful disorders. We are just the same when we have had a bad experience at the dentist for example. Many of my generation seem to have been treated by dentists trained in Nazi dental colleges, and bona fide phobias of dentists are commonplace. The newer generation of dentists are much more humane, ensuring that pain isn't automatically a part of dental therapy. Coupled with an improvement in dental health, this has meant that the younger generations have little fear of the dentists, and wonder what on earth their elders make such a fuss about. I am pleased to say that we as a practice have far fewer problems with pets who have been coming to us since puppy or kittenhood (or in some cases egghood), compared to patients we have inherited.

Remember your clients' feelings when coping with badly behaved pets. Don't lash out in retribution. This may take an iron discipline, particularly when you have a hamster or budgie firmly attached to your forefinger, but your local reputation will not be enhanced when little Cindy tells her classmates how the vet wildly shook her finger, resulting in Snuggles being propelled forcibly across the room, fortunately being prevented from landing in the car park by the window, which now has an interesting smear across it. Harsh words don't always go down well, even if warranted. I am well aware that it is galling to hear a client cooing 'Good boy Zeus, calm down', when Zeus has just tried to perform an amputation at the wrist. Perhaps it may seem that 'Sit down and behave Zeus you little *!?*!' is more appropriate, but the pet is not in a normal environment, and calming words are probably a better bet that confrontation in most cases.

Forewarned is forearmed. If a difficult case is coming in, be prepared. Perhaps tranquillizer tablets are the answer. Maybe the client should have the pet muzzled prior to entering the practice. If they practice the muzzling technique at home, getting the pet used to wearing one even in pleasant circumstances, then the pet won't immediately associate the sight of the muzzle with danger, pain and a telling off. Some pets are better handled by their owners. Many, I find, are far better if separated from their owners. Dogs and cats and birds sense their owners apprehension acutely, and react accordingly. They also gain confidence from proximity to their owners, leading them to be aggressive where they may not otherwise be so. Some dogs are hyperprotective of their owners, leading to conflict. Try taking the pet to a quiet room at the back of the practice where you and your nurse can try to examine and treat the patient in calmer surroundings. Many pets submit, and if not, you are freer to use firm tactics which, although legitimate, the owner may not fully appreciate. If nothing else at least the pet doesn't associate the owner with the unpleasant experience. If justified, use a sedative combination to make the experience more pleasant for owner, pet and vet. Several are available, and have varying degrees of efficacy.

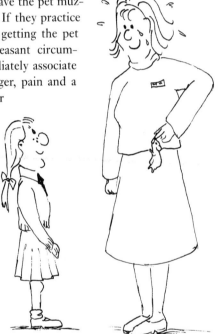

Many owners would rather that you conducted the less comfortable parts of your treatment out of their sight. They are a little squeamish when it comes to seeing their pet enfolded in a half-nelson with a tape tied raffishly around its muzzle and three members of staff dancing around giving conflicting instructions. This applies sometimes to procedures as seemingly mild as claw clipping. I would certainly advise against the practice of lancing that beautiful, juicy, ripe cat abscess in the consulting room. While we are doubtless under the impression that we are doing the client and pet a favour, reducing costs and avoiding anaesthetic fees, the owner simply sees a gleeful vet advancing on their precious cat, wielding a scalpel blade with a flourish and squeezing a glutinous fountain of richly coloured and odoured pus from the feline with the self-satisfied air of a conjurer producing an especially spectacular rabbit from a hat. Don't do it. It may be surprising, but your client will think you brutal and barbaric. The cat isn't bothered I know, but sadly the next time the owner puts her cat in a basket she won't be able to hear the cat going 'Hey! Let's go back to that Dr Lancer – he was fun!'.

Unrealistic promises

Although it is good to appear confident, and often comforting for the client if you give them an assurance, steer clear of making definite promises. We are dealing with living organisms. The beauty of these creatures is that no two are identical. No two examples of a disease that you see will replicate each other absolutely. It isn't uncommon for us to be contacted when a condition recurs and asked if there isn't some sort of guarantee, such as when their car was repaired. There are many possible answers to this provoking enquiry, starting with a discussion of how much it cost to repair their heap of metal. We have to be patient, however, and explain that the fact that the complaint has reappeared doesn't mean that we haven't performed our treatment correctly. What we must be careful of is making any sort of guarantee or promise which may turn out to be false.

There will be many occasions when you are keen to embark on a course of treatment which you have administered many times before, with perfect results, and yet the owner is reluctant. He has irrational fears about the drugs or the anaesthetic. He is worried about the financial outlay. He doesn't want to risk the pet becoming worse. You can do no more than reassure him as to the relative safety of the therapy, perhaps quoting the statistics of previous cases. Whatever you do, don't go all the way and say everything will be all right, the pet will survive the anaesthetic, the antibiotics won't harm it, the ear will definitely be better after surgery. Murphy's Law states that if only one in ten thousand cases won't go according to plan, it will be the one that you promised would be perfect.

You can soon learn to be persuasive and reassuring while being honest. I never shrink from telling the owners about the possible side effects of any treatment or procedure, and I may even add that those are only the ones we know about. The important point is the balance between the benefit that a patient will obtain from treatment set against the tiny chances of side effects or complications. The owner must be the one to decide, and to do that they should be in possession of the facts as you see them.

Avoiding telephone diagnosis

A few days experience in the consulting room will soon show you that even the most experienced pet owner sees clinical signs and their importance from a completely different viewpoint to your own. That should then lead you to vow to steer well clear of trying to make a diagnosis of any problem over the telephone, with only the owner's observations and opinion to guide you. Apart from their misinterpretations of symptoms, they will also put a slant on the presenting signs depending on their wishes. If they are desperate for you to climb out of bed at three in the morning, they will over dramatise, while if they can't be bothered to turn out, or are reluctant to splash out on an out-of-hours fee the pet will be 'comfortable' or 'not bothered'. You in turn will tend to guide them according to your state of mind, or your first thoughts as to a diagnosis. You may, for instance, however innocently, persuade yourself and the owner that a dog with signs of a gastric dilatation is suffering with indigestion, or that a cat with a gaping wound simply has a burst abscess.

This tendency for misunderstanding via the telephone can have amusing results. There was the miniature poodle which had 'a broken leg with the bone showing through the skin'. After rushing in to the surgery (on all fours), the dog underwent an emergency removal of polo mint from the fur of the front leg. The cat which had 'lost a leg', although there was no sign of blood, did at least come in on three legs. It was very relieved to have its front paw removed from its collar, where it had become wedged. The Persian cat which had given birth to a kitten which was hanging from its back end, but wouldn't allow anyone to touch it. This (neutered – honestly) cat proved to have a large, firm mat of fur hanging from its back end.

Another common source of misdiagnosis, by owners in most cases, leads me to a brief digression. I had the great pleasure of working with a locum from New Zealand some years ago. Let him be called Fred. We were all very fond of Fred, although he was a little eccentric. He once went swimming with his bleep on. He had the endearing habit of telling clients whose cats had abscesses in their paws that they had been afflicted by porcupine quills. Funnily enough, few clients questioned this interesting diagnosis. We his colleagues were mystified why this proved a popular diagnosis, since porcupines are not native to New Zealand. It turned out that Fred was getting them confused with hedgehogs, which he clearly considered hazardous little animals. I arrived back at work one Monday morning to find that Fred had spent much of the weekend wrestling with a frustrating case. A cat had been displaying signs of severe back pain. 'I've ruled out everything else,' said Fred 'so I have come down to a diagnosis of a trapped spinal nerve.' He certainly had ruled out most things. Blood tests, neurological exams, x-rays and even myelography had been employed to get to the bottom of the mystery. It felt cruel when Fred described the cat's presenting signs of loud yowling in pain, and rolling about on its back in agony to point out to him that it was a young entire female cat, which had simply come into season for the first time. Before condemning Fred, remember the vet's prayer: 'There, but for the grace of God, go I.' Fred certainly wasn't the first or the last vet to be taken in by a cat calling, but I think he probably ran up the largest bill for one.

Knowing when to refer

We all experience frustrating cases which seem to drag on and on. They may seem to respond to treatment temporarily but then relapse. A diagnosis may prove difficult to obtain. The owner may start to get restless. Inevitably in such cases we become a little stale. Having tried hard in the beginning to find a diagnosis or effective treatment, our judgement later on may be clouded by our fixation with one line of thinking. However much we try to avoid this, it is only to be expected. Once we have gone a certain way down one route, we may feel reluctant to suggest to the client that we should start again, or repeat large chunks of investigation.

There is no shame in seeking help with cases, whether at the beginning or well down the line. Clients won't usually deem you to be less competent because you want someone else's thoughts or advice. They know that everyone has different areas of expertise. Often simply having someone else looking at a case through fresh and unprejudiced eyes will allow a breakthrough. If nothing else, it is easier for a second vet to advise further tests or therapies rather than for you to appear to go back on your previous thinking.

By suggesting a second opinion before your client does, you will be able to, in the first instance, offer the client a chance to see someone else within your practice. This is good for the practice, and ensures that you will be backed up and supported fully. If it proves that expertise from outside the practice is required, then you can refer the client to a bona fide specialist. This is far better than the client simply upping sticks and heading down the road to your competition, who are no more expert than you are, and who, while remaining professional and uncritical, are unlikely to actually talk you up. You will also get your client back from a specialist, whereas they are less likely to return from your competition, even if they can do no better with the case than you. Finally, you have the opportunity to learn from the specialist's handling of the case, her diagnosis and treatment, which will stand you in good stead for the future.

I know that some vets are very loathe to refer cases, perhaps seeing referral as an admission of failure, or not wanting to lose control of the case. I feel that they and their clients and patients will be the losers from such an attitude. Know your limitations. Clients are completely used to being referred by their G P's as soon as they actually have anything wrong with them, so they are quite comfortable with the idea. Far better to jump before you are pushed.

Damage limitation

You are either incredibly careful and perfect or extremely fortunate if you progress through your career without any mistakes. Mistakes are going to happen. Hopefully they will all be minor ones, but some may be quite serious. Your method of handling them may prove of vital importance to your reputation.

Naturally my first piece of advice is 'Don't make any mistakes'. You should endeavour to avoid mistakes by being thorough and methodical. Develop routines for procedures and stick to them. Try to build in checks so that errors have to pass more than one set of eyes. For instance, lay staff should be trained to study which drugs they are dispensing rather than to automatically follow instructions. They may well pick up inappropriate prescriptions or errors of dosage before the medication reaches the client. They should be aware of anaesthetic protocols and question the vet if something unusual is taking place or being ordered. Try to avoid short cuts if they may compromise your performance. Double check treatment regimes that you are unfamiliar with. There are many ways for you to implement your own 'quality control'.

We must accept that some errors are going to slip through the net. How do we deal with these? If you have worked on developing a good client relationship, then you may find it easy to discuss such things with them. The vast majority of errors are small beer, causing no harm and soon put right. Some are more major. I don't wish to advise dishonesty, but it is possible not to draw a client's attention to a mistake. Often they are not aware that an error has occurred, or they may otherwise be unaware of how serious an error was. There is often an intense feeling of guilt which may make a vet feel like pouring out a confession and seeking forgiveness or censure. Be careful. Don't deny anything that you can't deny, but equally never make an admission of liability. Your professional indemnity insurers won't allow you to do this, just as you shouldn't admit liability in a car accident. It may often turn out that in fact a vet is not as liable as he or she thinks they are, and it is merely their guilt and disappointment which has made them feel that they are responsible.

I don't advise a certain economy with the truth lightly. I do so for several reasons. Firstly serious mistakes are very few and far between. I certainly don't know vets who make a habit of committing serious errors. We are all human, and if a mistake is a one off, we will feel bad enough without extra problems. Secondly you must ask whether it will help the client at all to know that an error has been made. They themselves will be feeling upset, possibly bereaved. If something could have been prevented, that will cause them more anguish. Thirdly, the trust and confidence that clients have in a vet is vital if the vet is to be able to minister to his patients effectively. I see no good in destroying that confidence unless it is truly justified. Clients would like to think of you as infallible, and you should try to live up to that.

Please don't think that I condone negligence or incompetence. From my experience these are truly rare. Negligent or incompetent practitioners probably deserve all they reap, but the conscientious, reliable and thorough vet who is the norm shouldn't be pilloried for suffering a stroke of bad luck.

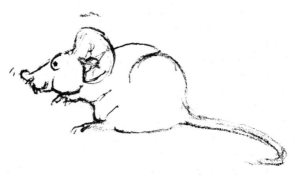

- The best way to look good is to avoid looking bad
- Older vets often command clients' respect – watch them to see why
- Good communication between staff is vital for a practice to look efficient
- Keeping clients well informed reduces misunderstandings, involves clients and makes them feel important
- Keep in touch – don't wait for clients to contact you
- You don't have to know everything, but you should 'know a man who does' and you should appear to know what you are doing
- Keep up to date with developments in veterinary science and current affairs – your clients will
- Be familiar with species and breeds of pet that are brought to you
- Clients will forgive much if they feel you genuinely care for your patients
- Send patients home after surgery looking clean, comfortable and with neat wounds
- Use the records as an *aide-mémoire* for personal details about pets and owners
- Be diplomatic when dealing with poorly behaved pets
- Don't perform seemingly gory procedures in front of clients
- Avoid telephone diagnosis
- Know your limitations – refer before a second opinion is sought

7

How to break bad news

Think of the client

An incident from her days of seeing practice is firmly lodged in the memory of a colleague. A couple of elderly ladies brought an elderly cat to see the vet. The cat had the classic signs of a severe pleural effusion. The vet promised to admit the cat and to carry out whatever investigations were necessary. The x-rays duly revealed a large thymic lymphoma with a profuse quantity of fluid in the chest, and very little lung tissue evident. When the cat recovered from its sedation, it was started on some therapy to alleviate the symptoms and replaced in its wicker basket. The elderly ladies duly returned, and the vet carried the basket and cat back to the consulting room to tell them about the findings. He explained what the problem was, stressed that it was incurable, outlined such palliative treatment as could be administered and finished by telling the clients that so serious was the condition that the cat could easily die at any moment. Having finished his summary of the case, he swung the cat basket onto the table in front of the now tearful ladies and opened the top, only to be confronted with an extremely dead cat. He hardly broke stride, but announced with a triumphant flourish 'See! I told you so!'

Clinical skill and surgical expertise are all very well, but what a client appreciates is bedside manner, and this is never more important than when they are receiving bad news. We must try to step back from a situation and see things from a client's viewpoint. When we have worked out that a pet is suffering from an interesting and challenging condition which is so rare that a practitioner might only expect to see one or two cases in a lifetime, don't expect your clients to share your sense of excitement and self-congratulation. Their pet is ill. The fact that the disease it is afflicted by is a candidate for 'disease of the year' at the local vet club is no compensation.

Our perceptions of the purpose of investigative procedures, and those of our clients differ fundamentally. When we perform blood tests, take x-rays, perform ecg's or ultrasound examinations, we seem to feel that we must turn up some abnormality to satisfy the client. As the results churn out of the biochemistry machine, the sight of an abnormally high blood chemistry figure may prompt a punching of the air and a sharp cry of 'Yesss!' The discovery of a mass in the chest on an x-ray leads to a big sigh of relief and a pleased nod of the head. We feel guilty going to contact the owner only to tell them that the tests have proved normal. Well here's something, guys. That's *good news*, OK? Put yourself in the pet's/client's position, and imagine that you were waiting for results of tests from the hospital, and imagine that they hadn't taken so long to be reported that you weren't already dead or had forgotten all about them. You'd like to hear that you had the all clear, wouldn't you? I know that if a patient is ill you and the client are hoping to discover the reason for it, but your investigations are presumably aimed at eliminating the nastier possibilities. When you do have an abnormality to report, don't impart the information in a manner which suggests that you are waiting for a pat on the back for being such a clever vet. Do so gently and appropriately.

Sympathising with owners

It helps greatly when trying to understand a client's feelings when they receive bad news if you have had some kind of similar experience. No one wishes ill fortune on any of you, but at some stage or another those of you who own pets will probably experience ill health, injury or loss of those pets. Make use of the feelings of loss, worry and concern when talking to owners. Talk to them about your own experiences and how they made you feel and how you coped with them.

Understanding that you have gone through similar experiences is quite a comfort to clients, and provides a useful bond between you. Knowing what courses of action you took and how you coped with your experiences helps them greatly.

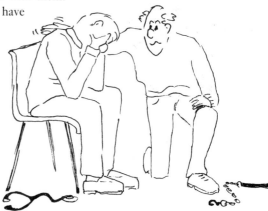

How much to tell and when to tell it

Clients have a right to know the facts relating to their pets. Apart from the fact that they own the animal concerned, they are also paying you for your attention. Veterinary science is somewhat imprecise in many ways, however. Who is to say what is fact and what is speculation? In many cases a definitive diagnosis is only to be obtained at post-mortem examination. You therefore control the information which is given to the owners, and you are able to put the slant that you choose upon that information. Massaging the information released may be done for many reasons: to make the vet look better or more competent, to spare the client's feelings, to buy time, to persuade the client to take a certain course of action. It isn't ethical to tell an actual untruth to a client, but you feel that there are times when it is justifiable to be economical with the truth. Be careful. Even with the best intentions in the world, subterfuge is a dangerous game. The client may not see things your way should he find that you haven't been entirely honest, or that you have kept important information back. It may seem unlikely that a client will discover such facts, but should a case not go according to plan and a second opinion be sought, your actions may well come to light.

It is better when you suspect that you have got bad news to report to a client, that you don't wildly speculate or give definite diagnoses to clients when you cannot possibly be sure that they are true. It is permissible to give your thoughts and differentials, but it may not be fair to upset a client before it is inevitable so to do. Even the most convincing evidence on a clinical examination can be quite misleading. For instance, I am sure that I am not alone in performing exploratory surgery on cats with abdominal masses, convinced that I was about to uncover an aggressive neoplasm, only to find a more benign problem such as an abscess, swollen lymph node or a treatable tumour. You may examine an animal with a history of moderately severe renal failure which appeared to have suddenly gone downhill with total anorexia, vomiting and dehydration. You may then, confident in your mind that the patient has descended into acute renal failure with a correspondingly bad prognosis, feel that you are saving the owner money and worry, the patient distress and yourself time if you present this to the owner as the diagnosis and recommend euthanasia. Without confirming your speculative diagnosis you may be missing a simple case of gastroenteritis, an unrelated infection or a foreign body. Give the owner bad news in at least two stages – voice your suspicions if need be, but give the really bad news when you are as sure as you are going to be that you are right.

There are some facts that clients don't need to be burdened with. First amongst these are the cases where a client has made a problem worse by their actions or lack of action. It is rare that a person will wilfully do harm to their pet. In other cases, only if it is going to serve some purpose, such as preventing a similar incident, is it necessary to torture clients by telling them the truth. If it does prove necessary to tell them, then it should be done gently and sympathetically, not in an accusing way. They feel bad enough that their pet is ill without being given an added burden of guilt. Clients may be slow to recognise symptoms or not appreciate their significance. They may have stopped giving the medication which you prescribed, or may have massively overdosed the pet. They may have decided to try home remedies or a faith healer before consulting you. They may have been too busy to bring the pet at the earliest opportunity. They may have been reluctant to call you out at night (it does happen). There are ways of informing them that they might have handled things differently without being too accusatory. Don't be self-righteous. We all do things that we perhaps would rather we hadn't as events unfold.

Clients may prefer to be spared the more unpleasant aspects of a pet's illness. They will feel more comforted if they think that their pet isn't in pain, or if it died in peace. Your job is to do your best to alleviate any suffering that the animal may experience, but you needn't make your clients fully aware of the grisly details. There is sometimes a temptation to talk a case up to make one's role in it more significant. This really isn't necessary, and if the patient hasn't recovered it may simply be cruel.

There may have been decisions and choices that you or the clients failed to make during the course of a disease. Sometimes had you done things differently, the outcome may conceivably have been altered. These are important factors for you as the clinician to consider, as they will form an important part of your experience, building up a useful database for you to call on when confronted with a similar problem. It isn't important for a client to agonise over these wrong turnings and missed opportunities. There is little point in discussing them, for who can say what might have happened if between you, you had followed another course of action? Do all you can to reassure the client that they did the best they could for their pet.

The gloomy approach

There is a body of opinion that suggests that clients should always be presented with a worst case scenario when embarking on a course of treatment. After all, if the worst comes to the worst, the client is forewarned, and if the patient improves the vet has helped it through against the odds. Although taking this approach will rarely let you down, it hardly inspires confidence in the owner and doesn't put you in the best light. It may even lead to the owners not embarking on therapy, or not following it through as they are already depressed about the outcome.

There are some situations and conditions where this approach may be justified, although it should be moderated. Many vets have a conditioned reflex when a canary is brought into the consulting room. Almost before they greet the client, they find themselves saying 'I should warn you that some canaries will find the stress of handling too much and may expire'. A similar approach is often taken when dealing with birds of all other sorts: 'Of course, by the time you notice that a bird is unwell, it is usually already seriously ill, so we can't expect too much from our treatment'. These 'truths' may have a degree of accuracy, but I can honestly say that I have never had a canary drop dead on me just from the stress of examination, and it is actually possible to treat birds very effectively, assuming that you haven't put the client off completely.

It may be worth taking a pessimistic line when embarking on treatment of chronic conditions such as otitis and dermatoses, if only to bring home to clients that they are not the simple conditions that they may appear to be. Clients who seem to be blithely unaware of the seriousness of their pet's condition may need a hefty dose of pessimism to alert them to the possibility that there may not be a happy ending. I can recall several occasions when I have discovered a potentially life threatening condition necessitating surgery. Having explained (as I thought) the situation to the client, persuaded them of the need for urgent surgery and perhaps even got them to sign for permission for euthanasia if all hasn't gone well, they have nodded seriously then asked me to be sure and clip the pet's claws or empty its anal sacs while under the anaesthetic.

The eternal optimist

The opposite approach to the pessimist's is to be airily unconcerned about the potential complication of a disorder and its therapy. To have boundless reserves of confidence which will sweep a client along with you. To break bad news in one breath but to soften the blow with your assurances that you can overcome the problems.

Clients will initially take to this approach. Why not, when the optimist is telling them what they want to hear? The trouble is that the optimism is all too often misplaced, and all that is happening is that the truly bad news is being delayed. Sometimes this approach is taken because the vet feels unable to give the harsh facts to the client. She would rather put off the evil moment until it is inevitable, or maybe a colleague will have taken the responsibility. Unfortunately, it is better to take a more honest approach, giving the true facts of the case and the likely outcome, even if the vet is then upbeat about the chances of treatment. The eternal optimist is likely to have to let a lot of clients down gently as the cases progress.

It is useful to be upbeat about certain conditions and procedures where clients tend to be rather reluctant and gloomy themselves. General anaesthesia in older animals is one area where clients show great hesitation. Without being unrealistic in my promises, I would say to clients that I wouldn't make age a reason for avoiding general anaesthesia. Dental treatment is another procedure which may take some persuasion. You can give clients a very positive prognosis if they will consent to treatment. The trick is not to be over the top in your predictions, even if you are desperate to persuade the client to go ahead for the sake of the pet. Be as positive as you like, provided that you point out the possible complications, and you are fairly sure that you are not going to let your clients down with a bump.

The gentle approach

Whatever the item of bad news you are having to impart to a client, whether it be confirmation of a diagnosis, an unexpected complication or a fatality, be sure to handle them gently. It is possible in a busy working environment to have to rush too much when giving owners information. This can make you appear callous, even if it is untrue. As ever, remember that the client isn't aware of your workload, the queue of people waiting to see you or the other calls you have to make. When you are speaking to her, she expects a calm one-to-one conversation with all of your attention. If unpleasant information is involved, it is necessary to take your time. Be ready to answer any queries. Allow the client time to come to terms with what you have just told them. If it is very bad news, and they seem somewhat shocked, offer to call them later, or to speak to them if they call when they are ready.

It is all too easy to forget that something that to us is a routine problem, or a disorder which is eminently treatable may seem catastrophic to our clients. This may be because they don't understand the details of the problem, they are worried about the cost or they have had a previous pet with the disorder, or know of a friend's pet which had it. Be sensitive when imparting information. We may airily classify a mass in the skin or internally as a tumour. To the average client this is a very emotive and upsetting word. They may have relatives who have suffered from cancer. Even if we are quite sure that the growth is a tumour, we should either be very circumspect in how we communicate this to our client, or hold back from making pronouncements until we have confirmed our diagnosis. There is a fine line to walk between completely shielding a client from the possibilities that a condition is serious, even life threatening, and causing them undue and perhaps unnecessary worry. Only practice will guide you in this, but a softly, softly approach is usually kinder.

It is not uncommon for a patient to be brought in for a routine procedure such as a booster vaccination, and for a serious disorder to be detected at that time. A classic example is an elderly cat which proves on examination to have a large and probably malignant abdominal tumour palpable. Again, bear in mind the devastating effect that this is likely to have on the client. Don't whoop with excitement at your excellent diagnostic skill. Don't callously inform the client that if you were they, you wouldn't bother with the inoculation. Carefully inform them that you have found an abnormality which may prove to be serious, but that you should look into it before making a definitive statement. Do be honest. It isn't fair to lead a client to believe that your findings don't suggest a major problem, or that the disorder will lend itself to therapy if you then completely reverse this opinion later on. They will appreciate your honesty and a frank discussion of the possibilities. I would merely suggest that you do offer a range of possibilities rather than going straight for the jugular.

Clients will respond to bad news in a variety of ways, which you may find distressing, confusing, worrying or hard to believe in your early days in practice. They may respond with disbelief, anger at you, denial, guilt, apparent indifference or complete breakdown. They may be embarrassed at showing their emotions in front of a stranger. They may have

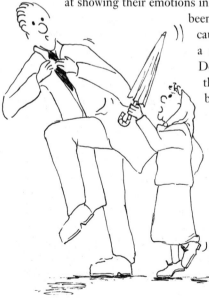

been unaware that such an event could cause them distress. You must provide a sympathetic and encouraging ear. Don't act embarrassed in your turn at their discomfiture. Owners should be free to let their feelings show at such an emotional time. Let them know that it is all right to be upset and to shed a tear. Say soothing things. Don't stand back as though you are an observer. This is a particularly hard area for young vets to deal with, having not had much experience of comforting distraught owners, and yet it is important for us to show compassion and empathy with our clients. Try to find calm surroundings away from the hustle and bustle of the practice to talk to the client. Offer them a seat. Perhaps a cup of tea. Anything to ease the pain of the facts they must absorb.

Clients may seek confirmation in terms of a second opinion from one of your colleagues. In this case, whatever you do, do not get on your high horse and take umbrage. Your colleague will back you up, and it is entirely understandable for the client to want confirmation of what you are telling them. I am only surprised that more do not seek such corroboration. Seeking a colleague's opinion yourself is one way of helping the owner to come to terms with what you are telling them.

However the rest of your handling of a case goes, the clients will remember the way in which you dealt with them at a time of great stress and worry. No matter how the case goes, if you have been sympathetic, helpful and provided the client with a shoulder to lean on, you will earn their respect and gratitude.

Do your own dirty work

Clients far prefer to have one vet attending to each condition that affects their pet, rather than having a succession of vets performing each stage of the diagnosis and treatment. They don't like speaking to different vets about the case, having to repeat details over and over. They like to know that one vet has the pet's condition fresh in his mind. This is surely the ideal for us as veterinarians as well. We must feel a sense of duty to the patient and owner, and an interest in following the case through to its conclusion. The time when we may be tempted to pass a case on is when it is not likely to go too well. When the time comes to admit that we cannot go any further, that we have discovered that the case is untreatable, or that a more complicated course of treatment is necessary, or that we are having to revise our original diagnosis. How easy it would be to allow another vet to pick up the case, liase with the owner and carry on, while we put it out of our mind and concentrate on something a little easier or more rewarding.

Unfortunately we do have a responsibility. We must be strong and honest enough to pass on bad news as well as good to our clients. Far better to hear of complications from the vet that the client is familiar with. You will be able to clarify items that the client is unsure of. You are in the best position to review the case and explain the next course of action to be taken. You should have built up a certain rapport with that client and demonstrated that you genuinely care for his pet.

If you have to break bad news, it is far preferable to communicate in person with the client if at all possible. Failing this, be sure that it is you who contact them by telephone to pass on the information. Don't leave details of unpleasant findings on an answerphone – rather ask the client to contact you later. Don't leave a colleague, or even worse a member of the lay staff, to do your dirty work for you. This may happen inadvertently if you have been unable to reach a client, and when they phone the practice a receptionist or nurse may read from the records that the dog has terminal liver failure, the cat has F I V or the hamster's rectal prolapse is out again. Take steps to avoid this happening.

After you have delivered your unwelcome news, or while a difficult case is progressing, make yourself available for the client. This may mean that you are prepared to speak to clients from home on your days off or after hours. It means being sure to return their calls when they want to speak to you. Be there for them. They need a source of stability and authority to help them through, and an understanding ear.

Body language

It is worth making a little study of people that you admire or dislike. Observe the way that they bear themselves when dealing with situations. As much as the words that they say, their body language has an influence on the way we feel about them, and how successful they are in getting their message across. The right posture and gestures and we feel that the speaker is being open and truthful, is confident, is comfortable with our presence. Someone else may seem shifty, worried, as though they have something to hide. A third may come across as overbearing, bullying and trying to force their point of view.

Your body language when dealing with clients is important as well. To a certain extent you must learn to act with your body, to give a confident and trustworthy performance, even when you are unsure of yourself, worried about a client's reaction to what you are telling them or experiencing feelings of frustration or possibly anger towards them. Not always easy to do, particularly when you are starting out in practice, giving advice to clients far older than you are, or who have been keeping and breeding dogs or cats since before you were a little zygote. If you want to be trusted and taken seriously, liked even, you must master the lingo.

To some, confident body language comes naturally. Some individuals are naturally assured, comfortable with themselves. Even to those fortunates I would say take care lest you seem too cocksure. Aim for positive not cocky, sympathetic not callous and open rather than shifty.

Hold your head up and face the client. Be erect, don't slouch or lean all over the place. Never sit while talking to a client, unless you have sat them down first. Don't cross your arms, an often involuntary gesture which makes one seem closed and defensive. Talk to the client clearly. Don't mumble to the table or your feet, and avoid talking to them while you are facing away from them. Don't let them talk to your back – if they start while you are turned away, stop what you are doing and turn back again. Don't be afraid of physical contact if they want it (but only if they want it). Many people will wish to shake your hand after a successful conclusion to a case, or even an unsuccessful conclusion, as a gesture of thanks. Take their hand confidently. Wear an appropriate expression when talking to people, if only to show that you are paying attention to what they are saying. Smile if possible. I know the job can be serious and heart-breaking, but it can also be tremendous fun. Try to avoid adopting postures which seem dismissive or disrespectful of clients.

When breaking bad news, or discussing the details of worrying cases with owners, maintain your confident posture, even when commiserating. However unintentionally, you may give the client the idea that you are hiding something from her or that you feel guilty for some reason if you cannot look her in the eye as you discuss her case. Maintain an open and honest stance, inviting questions. Don't keep your distance, delivering your findings from the far end of the room. Move towards the client, indicating that you and she are in partnership in trying to help her pet or decide its future. In short adopt poses with clients much like the ones you would adopt with your friends.

When things go wrong

There are unfortunately going to be many times when events haven't gone according to plan. These may range from simple errors such as forgetting to dispense some treatment to mislaying a blood sample before it reaches the laboratory, to serious errors which affect the health of your patient or your client's pocket. It is a little futile to advise you to avoid such errors as they will happen occasionally regardless. You should be able to minimise them, however, by attention to detail and good communication between you, your colleagues, your lay staff and the client.

If you are fortunate, most of your errors will go unnoticed, doing no harm to man nor beast. Those mistakes which are noticed will affect the whole range of clients, from those angelic souls who are willing to forgive and forget anything, to professional complainers always with an eye to what they can get out of a situation. By cultivating good client relations, proving yourself to be normally reliable and diligent and having a pleasant, likeable manner you will improve the odds of the client being on your side if an error occurs.

Unless the error is minor and will cause no problems, in which case thank your lucky stars and learn from the experience, it is best to point out minor problems such as forgetting to check a sample or clipping up the wrong leg before an operation to the client as soon as possible. Explain what has happened and what steps you will take to rectify the situation. Apologise profusely for small errors. If you have done something a little more drastic, like cutting off the wrong leg after clipping it, errors which may affect the reputation of the practice or lay it open to action, consult the principal or partners immediately for advice. They may take the matter out of your hands and handle the client themselves. Depending on the seriousness of the matter it may be necessary to contact the practice's professional indemnity insurers, who will advise on the correct procedure. If you are left to contact the client be direct, as honest as prudence allows and be humble and apologetic. I would advise practices to be flexible about fees in cases affected by errors or omissions, but in these days of litigation one should be careful not to make any admission of liability and to make plain that waiving or reducing of fees is a gesture of goodwill rather than an acceptance of guilt.

Anaesthetic deaths

There can be few more harrowing experiences for clients and veterinary staff than unexpected anaesthetic deaths. The tremendous feelings of guilt and disappointment are compounded by a sense of dread at having to tell the owner of the incident and an anticipation of their angry response. Modern anaesthetic regimes and drugs have helped to reduce these unfortunate losses, but you are going to have to face up to several incidents during the course of your career.

Anaesthetic deaths take two forms. There are the deaths in high-risk patients, usually older pets or pets with already diagnosed disorders which might affect their ability to withstand a general anaesthetic. It might still be justifiable to include exotic pets in this category, as although modern anaesthetics have also made their chances of surviving anaesthesia much greater, they still experience higher levels of stress and problems of hypothermia and dehydration more severely than cats and dogs. The owners of these patients should not be allowed to be unaware of the risks of anaesthesia. Without wishing to put them off having beneficial surgeries performed, they should be clear about the possibility of something going wrong.

More devastating by far are those cases where a pet, seemingly in fine health, dies during a routine procedure such as spaying or castration. I am not going to lecture you on how to keep risks to a minimum – never assuming an animal is healthy without checking it first, not allowing your attention to wander while a patient is asleep, using a safe anaesthetic regime rather than a convenient or cheap one. Even the most cautious vet will lose a few patients which seemed to be practically no risk at all.

These are the cases where the clients will be bewildered and angry at losing their pet. They may feel guilt at having booked the pet in for the procedure in the first place. They are likely to experience feelings of anger and betrayal that you have allowed this to happen. They will certainly want to know why and how it could occur. They are often upset because they feel that their pet has been taken from them without them being present or having a chance to say goodbye.

Do whatever you can to ensure that such an event doesn't come as a complete surprise to a client. No doubt before admitting a high-risk patient you will have explained the dangers of anaesthesia in such a case. As the average client's perception of the risks of general anaesthesia is far more gloomy than our own, owners of these pets may be more surprised when you tell them that their patient has survived than if you should have to inform them of a death. For more routine operations, ensure that your practice has clear consent forms which point out that all surgical procedures carry risks. Staff admitting pets should be sure that the client has read the form before signing it. If they have forgotten their glasses, for instance, staff should read the form to them. Don't fail to take a contact phone number which will actually be of some use during the day. Be honest with clients when discussing surgery with them. Don't belittle the chances of something going wrong in order to persuade the client to go ahead. The decision to go ahead with a procedure under general anaesthesia must be the client's, however strong your advice.

If a patient has died, first consult a partner or senior colleague for guidance. Your practice may have set guidelines for such cases. One of the partners may feel that it is their place to contact the owner to pass on the bad news. They may want to ascertain the full details and circumstances before informing the client.

In an ideal world we would tell the client about their loss face to face. In practice we will usually be communicating with them by means of the telephone. Apart from gathering the facts of the case as mentioned above, there shouldn't be any delay in informing the client. Do not allow the client to call the practice to find out about their pet's progress, only to be told of the tragedy. This makes the practice look inefficient and callous. Whatever the reaction of the client, you should be gentle, sympathetic, apologetic (without implying that you have done anything wrong) and prepared to answer any questions, many of which may be illogical or even insulting. In a time of great stress for you as well as the client, you must not be over defensive or confrontational, however the client speaks to you. They have a good reason to be upset and act irrationally, whereas you do not. In almost all cases clients amaze me by their understanding and generosity. This is helped by working hard to build a good and trusting relationship with them. Often they are consoling the vet by the end of the conversation. You must expect the worst sort of reactions as well, however and control your responses so as not to inflame a delicate situation. By being open, convincing the client that you are not hiding anything, and being prepared to fully and frankly discuss the case later when they have overcome the initial shock, you will retain the trust of almost all clients.

Most owners will want to know why such a thing has happened. Being strictly honest, you may not really know in most cases what has been the cause of death. You should have a presentable theory to offer the client, though. There is no need to present it as gospel truth, but simply as the most likely hypothesis. Offer an autopsy, either to be performed at your practice, by you or one of your colleagues, or at an independent practice. Offer to see the client whenever convenient to go over the case in detail. Contact them with a letter a day or so later expressing your condolences.

Such occurrences are very stressful to all veterinary surgeons, and to young ones in particular. Remember that, provided you have been operating correctly, these deaths are not your fault. They will occur to the most cautious anaesthetist from time to time. Thankfully modern anaesthetics and protocols reduce the numbers of anaesthetic deaths all the time. Don't fear that you will lose the faith of your clients. A case which happened to me some years ago always springs to mind. A client booked two bitches in to be spayed, a mother and daughter. We chose the younger bitch to begin with, and tragically she died virtually as we injected the intravenous anaesthetic agent. She was unresponsive to our efforts at resuscitation. With heavy heart I called the owner. He immediately assumed that it was the older bitch that had died, and was quite philosophical. On learning that it was in fact the young bitch which had succumbed he was rather shocked. Assuming that he wouldn't want us to proceed I asked him when he wanted to collect the mother. 'When she's recovered from spaying, of course!' he replied. He was most insistent that I should operate on the second bitch. Although it was perhaps one of the most uncomfortable operations that I have performed, I have never ceased to be grateful to that client for the faith and trust that he showed in us. Be upset, be remorseful, but remember that you are not a worse vet for the (very) occasional anaesthetic death.

The bill

The normal bill

We are very poor as a profession at recognising our worth. We tend to try and forget about the financial side of our job as far as possible. We should be proud that we are able to provide ever improving standards of medical and surgical care to our patients, and that we retain a reputation for high standards of patient and client care, and commitment to our calling. This is recognised by our clients, and yet there may be complaints about the high charge of veterinary fees. Those same clients are willing to part with far larger sums of money to other service providers who they are fully aware do not provide the same expertise or care that the veterinary profession does. The situation is not helped by the fact that there is a National Health Service which appears to provide free health care. In fact the average taxpayer pays out a large proportion of his income to fund the National Health Service. Most people pay in far more than they will ever take out, but they remain blissfully unaware of this.

You might ask them to compare the cost of veterinary attention with private medical costs, which would be a fairer comparison. For similar treatments, the vet is able to charge a mere fraction of the hospital's fee. You might also point out that we are able to provide life saving surgery for an amount less than the cost of the weekly shopping bill. How does their bill compare to their last car service? Compare the cost of consulting a vet with consulting a plumber or electrician. Are they suggesting that a vet is less qualified and therefore less valuable than these service providers? Is a living organism less complex than a tap, a cistern or a boiler?

Don't be embarrassed or coy about your bills. Present them confidently and be assured that you are giving value for money. Don't be apologetic or whistle in a shocked manner as the invoice is printed out. Most clients are quite prepared to pay a fair price for a good job. Always soften the blow for clients by providing them with a guide as to the costs of procedures before they go ahead with them. If they are forewarned of the rough amounts that they are dealing with, then it is up to them to decide whether or not they can afford to proceed. Be diligent about keeping the client up to date with costs, and let them know if the bill is going to rise significantly above your original guideline. In short, don't keep the bill as a big surprise to be unveiled as they collect their pet from you. Clients are happy to pay for your services as long as they are kept informed.

The bill when something has gone wrong

Ah. Tricky. There are many factors to take into consideration when calculating the bill for a procedure which hasn't quite gone according to plan. If the error is due to a mistake by the practice, clearly the client can't be charged for the mistake, and the practice may well have to be prepared to lose a little money to put things right or soothe the client. Money well spent if the client is happy at the end of the day. Remember that a disgruntled client may well moan to all who will listen about his bad experience. If the practice has manifestly done all it can to rectify the error, the publicity you gain may well prove to be good rather than damaging.

If things have not gone perfectly through no direct fault of the practice, it is harder to determine the correct course of action. I am not really discussing the run-of-the-mill case where patients seem to resist all efforts to get them better, or where they do their best to hide the diagnosis from the veterinary surgeon. This is just life, and if we only charged properly for completely successful cases they would have to be very expensive in order to provide the practice with sufficient income. The problematical cases are those where perhaps the patient has died, or surgery to correct a problem has not been successful or a problem has recurred where it would not reasonably have been expected to do so. Here again practices will have established procedures to follow.

Taking the worst scenario first, it would seem churlish and insensitive to expect clients to pay for cases of unexpected anaesthetic death. If your practice is going to ask you to seek payment from the owners then I wouldn't know what advice to give you (seek a new practice?). For cases of death in higher-risk patients, you will often have invested quite some time and effort in the patient before it succumbs, and you are quite justified in seeking payment for this. Not to charge, although a generous gesture, may plant the idea that you are somehow feeling guilty. Do consider the client's feelings when presenting the invoice. It is not a good idea to press for payment while they are trying to cope with the loss of their pet. Be prepared to wait.

In other cases where things have not proceeded ideally, yet you have not made actual mistakes, it is again reasonable to expect payment. It is important to stress to clients through this that you are not at fault and it is merely circumstances that have conspired to bring about a disappointing result.

It would seem sensible for a practice to take a flexible view of pricing when all has not gone as well as it should have. A reasonable, fair price should be expected by a client, whereas charging top whack may produce an indignant response and stir up trouble. If clients are told when any price reductions are given, it should be pointed out that they are purely a goodwill gesture lest they be taken as compensation or evidence of wrongful practice.

- Try to see things from the client's perspective
- Tailor your level of pessimism or confidence to each case and client
- Don't let clients down with a bump
- Don't delegate the task of giving bad news
- Be honest about most mistakes, and have a plan for rectifying them ready
- Discuss your practice's policy on serious errors or anaesthetic deaths before they happen
- The practice is entitled to payment even when the outcome of a case hasn't been ideal, but it is sensible to be sympathetic when charging

---

8

Awkward situations

When you start in practice you may feel overwhelmed by the clients, the workload, the other staff, the practice protocol. You may feel that every consultation represents an awkward situation. Hopefully you will be working in a practice which has well established methods of working and a uniform approach to clients and to dealing with cases. Such a well ordered environment allows you to slip into the routine of working easily, and ensures good and consistent support from veterinary and lay staff. There are always some situations which will prove to be a little trickier to handle than others, because they offer potential for embarrassment or misunderstanding or recrimination, or they may land you in trouble however unintentionally.

Second opinions 1: to you

All graduates, older as well as younger, would be well advised to read their *Guide to Professional Conduct* from time to time and attempt to abide by its principles. They would also do well to bear in mind the useful adage 'deal with others as you would be dealt with'.

You will be confronted regularly with cases which are second opinions from other practices. You will have the advantage when dealing with these cases of knowing how the case has unfolded so far, what the results of investigations so far are, what treatment has been given and which was successful. You will also have a client who, having thrown her lot in with you, is more likely to follow your advice and allow for extra expenditure.

With all these advantages you can afford to be generous about your predecessor. As Billy Wilder said, hindsight has twenty-twenty vision. Don't be too full of your own importance if you manage to improve the pet's condition. Always treat colleagues with professional courtesy. Follow established procedures for informing the first vet when a second opinion is sought with you. Often the clients will be reluctant to divulge the name of the previous vet. They may be worried how she will react when she finds out that her client isn't satisfied. They may not feel that the vet has done anything wrong, but they wish to get a fresh batch of ideas. They may even be intending to return to the practice and don't want to sour relations. You need to coax the information out of them. Apart from your obligations of professional courtesy, you should explain to the clients that it is in their own interests for you to be familiar with all the details of the case so far. You can then make use of previous test results, and avoid suggesting useless courses of action or treatment, saving the clients time and money and hopefully bring about a resolution more rapidly. You yourself will have the benefit of any details that the clients have been unable to reveal to you, or facts which they misunderstood and thus misled you with. Technically you should not really see the case if the clients won't tell you who they have been seeing, but I suppose that there is nothing to make them reveal that they have already seen a vet, however obvious it may be to you.

Make no criticism, actual or implied, of the original veterinary surgeon, however the case seems to have been handled. Apart from being defamatory, it would also mean you decrying a vet when you have only heard one side of the story. After all, many second opinions are sought simply because of misunderstandings between the vet and client. The clients have often got hold of entirely the wrong end of the stick, not always through their own fault, I might add. The practice which fails to communicate well with its clients and which fails to explain themselves well is destined to lose many clients who will seek the help of more understanding vets. Remember also than second opinions are a two way process – your neighbouring practice will probably receive clients from you who are not entirely satisfied with your handling of their pet's health. If you are consistently ethical and uncritical about your competition, they will repay the service.

If you examine the pet and the details of the history and come to the conclusion that the original vet has done all that she could and you would not reasonably be able to improve on the case, you should offer the client an opportunity to return to their first practice. They will often be reluctant to do this as they may feel awkward about having sought a second opinion in the first place, or because they have lost faith in the first practice.

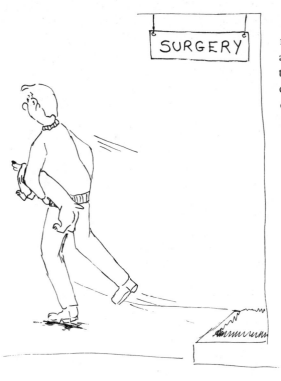

SURGERY

In many cases a second opinion is sought more because of the attitude of the practice than because the client doubts their clinical acumen. Once you have established that you will continue to see the client, it is courteous to inform the first practice, together with any further diagnosis you may have made. It is helpful, if not always appreciated, if you pass on any criticisms the client may have about the handling of the case, so that the original practice may at least know why it has lost a client. It is far preferable for the practices in a neighbourhood to be on good terms and able to communicate with each other in this way, rather than literally treating each other as competition and trying to score points off one another. Ultimately that will not improve the image of veterinary practice in your area.

Second opinions 2 : from you

No one is perfect, sadly. However diligent and thorough and knowledge-able you are, there will be cases which do not progress smoothly. You may also be presented with conditions which are unusual and perhaps best dealt with by practitioners with more experience in the particular field. The skill here is to be able to detect firstly when you are beginning to flounder, and secondly when the clients are beginning to get a little restless. Clients are often very reluctant to question you to your face, and if you are not careful the first you may know of their discontent is when your neighbouring practice calls you to inform you that a second opinion is being sought.

By being the one to suggest a second opinion, you can remain in control of the case. To begin with, there may be a colleague in your practice who has the required expertise. Even if no one specialises in the area you are dealing with, a fresh mind may spot something you have missed or be able to suggest a different approach. If no one inside the practice can help further, then you can arrange for the pet to be referred to a bona fide expert. This benefits you as you will retain the client, and hopefully learn something about dealing with similar cases, and it benefits the client, who would otherwise seek the opinion of another general practitioner who may well not even possess your level of expertise in this area.

Clients will not think any the worse of you if you are the one to suggest that a more expert opinion is required. They are often tickled pink that their pet requires a specialist. As with many situations in life, have the common sense to know when to jump before you are pushed.

If a client should seek a second opinion before you suggest it, you may be lucky enough to have one that asks you first. Don't take umbrage. Discuss with the client why it is that they would like to see someone else. You may well be able to sort things out with them and reassure them that everything necessary is being done. As ever, good communication is vital. You should discuss the progress of a case regularly with the client, together with your future treatment plans, so that they know that you do actually have a plan. If they still want the second opinion, offer to refer them to a suitable veterinarian. If you first find that a client wants a second opinion when another vet calls you up, be helpful and pass on case histories with good grace. If you feel that the problem has been one of misunderstanding, you might write to the client and explain your point of view. Never try to make the client feel bad about seeking another opinion, and try to maintain a good relationship with them. In this way you will leave open the opportunity for them to return to your practice if they should so desire at a later date.

Serial clients

A variation on the second opinion theme are the serial clients. These are clients who habitually drift from one practice to another, for one of a variety of reasons. They may see a different practice for each condition that their pet develops. They may continually become disgruntled after a few visits to each clinic and move on in search of different scenery. They may simply be habitual debtors who outstay their welcome. Most annoying are those who see one practice during the day, but call upon the more convenient one out of hours.

These are not quality clients that the practice should strive to retain and foster. Their approach to healthcare for their pets makes it impossible to develop a good relationship with them. They are less likely to be committed in terms of seeking the best of care for their animals. The best approach to these clients is to explain that in order for the practice to develop a relationship with them, and in order that their pets can receive the top quality healthcare they deserve, they need to decide upon one practice to use and to stick with it. They should not be encouraged into the practice for the sake of a quick buck when they want some flea treatment or a booster.

Out-of-hours calls

Perhaps the most unpopular part of a vet's working life is the portion spent on duty. Even when the duty is quiet, there is the constant threat hanging over one of a telephone call, which may signify anything from a torn claw to a gastric torsion or caesarean destined to keep one up all night. The annoyance can be aggravated by some clients' tendency to sit on problems for days until they becomes desperately urgent at half past eleven on a Friday night. Some clients also seem to treat the out-of-hours service as a higher price, but more convenient service for which they are quite happy to pay a premium.

One vet was called at around midnight by a gentleman who asked him if he knew anything at all about rabbits. Bristling somewhat, the vet replied in the affirmative. 'Oh good,' said the man. 'What do you call a male rabbit?' After the somewhat exasperated vet had answered the question, the man thanked him profusely. 'My wife's doing the crossword, and she won't let me get to sleep until she's finished.'

Another story, no doubt apocryphal, although the source swears it is true, concerns a vet who was called out at the weekend to see a desperately ill terrier. On arriving at the house he was greeted by a lady and a very lively and obviously well dog. In reply to his query, the woman informed him that she was very sorry, but her washing machine wasn't working and the vet's call-out fee was much cheaper than the plumber's.

I have had a call from someone in the early hours who has been concerned because he was looking at his fish and thought it was a bit depressed. Why on earth would you examine your fish at 3 a.m.? Others have called for advice when their bitch was whelping, and then happily called back every twenty minutes to report each perfectly normal delivery of a perfectly normal puppy, clearly under the impression that I wouldn't get to sleep until I knew that the whole litter was out and healthy. (Well, they were right there, weren't they?) A couple who lived about 15 miles to the east of the surgery called at about 10 p.m. in a great panic from a phone box. They were on holiday and the dog had cut its leg badly. They were packing up and heading back immediately from Wales (150 miles to the west of the surgery) and would meet me back at their house. The phone was down before I could get a word in. Why not find a local vet, or at least have the sense to come to the surgery? We should be flattered that our clients are willing to travel such distances to see us, I suppose.

If you are to be happy in your working life, you must try to get used to being on duty, and even to learn to relax. I know vets who tell me that they have trouble sleeping at night if they are on call, always anticipating the phone ringing. There is no doubt that time spent on call is an annoyance. It needs to be done, however, and it is the time when you will have to exercise your best client handling skills. If we provide a twenty-four hour service, something the profession is rightly proud of, we mustn't make clients feel bad for using it. They can be gently educated so that they don't take the service for granted, and have some consideration for the vets. It can be stressed to them that it is a service for genuinely urgent cases. They shouldn't, however, be discouraged from calling us until the very last moment. Far better that they should call us at an early stage of their pet's illness and receive useful advice than to wait until only drastic action is going to help.

You, on the end of the telephone, are not really in a position to determine how serious a pet's condition is. If a client chooses to exaggerate, and you end up seeing a pet which could quite happily have waited until the following morning, surely this is far better than you persuading a client that the patient isn't as bad as they think, and finding that the pet is seriously ill or dead on the morrow. Even if a condition isn't strictly an emergency, the pet is often in discomfort. If you are able to provide relief from suffering, then surely you should be prepared to do so.

Always be polite to clients, whatever the circumstances of the call. Clients may often seem rude, abrupt, demanding and insensitive to your discomfort. Remember that they are usually upset that their pet is not well, and their behaviour is not normal. Make allowances. I have often found myself driving to the surgery in a disgruntled state of mind, cursing the client and his pet roundly and calculating how I can bump up the bill to the sort of level that might provide some small measure of compensation. By the time I reach the surgery and see the pet being brought in I have usually regained my equanimity, and by the end of the consultation I am likely to be trying to keep the bill to the lowest legitimate figure that I can manage. Just as it is often more enjoyable to travel in expectation than to arrive, the anticipation of being called in to the surgery is often the most irritating thing about being on call. The cases that you see are often more interesting after all, and you are usually able to make a real difference to the pet . If you are able to be polite and calm when seeing clients out of hours, you will rise greatly in their estimation.

Be careful never to refuse to see a patient out of hours. As we have said, you cannot tell via the telephone how necessary it is to see a patient. Always offer to see the animal. Let the client decide whether or not it is vital for you to see them. The out-of-hours surcharge is the deciding factor. Let the client know how much it is going to cost to see their pet, and let them decide whether or not the pet's condition warrants it. Accepting that emergency cover can be abused in some areas, and that the costs and inconvenience of proving 24-hour cover are not compensated whatever the surcharges might be, I am not a fan of making surcharges enormous simply to discourage clients from calling vets out. They should be realistic. High enough to make a client seriously consider the gravity of the condition. Charges should not be punitive, a way of getting some malicious satisfaction out of the affair.

Visits

A day or two after I joined a practice, I was preparing to go on a visit to a local housing estate. Let's call it Shangri-La. As I gathered my equipment, one of the nurses told me a cheering story. When she and her husband moved to the area, he got a job with the local dairy as a milkman. On his first day he and his new colleagues moved from the dairy building into the compound where the milk floats were charging their batteries. His round happened to take in Shangri-La. As he walked down the line, various milkmen hopped into their floats. Approaching the end of the queue of floats, he still hadn't found his. At the end of the line his float appeared – the only one out of about twenty-four to be enclosed in a wire cage, 'in case of high jinks' as the foreman said. Having delivered this tale, the nurse declined my invitation to accompany me and busied herself elsewhere.

There are several reasons why visits are not popular. They take up an inordinate amount of time. In some cities they may involve rather too much opportunity to study traffic flow, or lack of it. In some areas it is simply not considered safe for one member of staff to go out on a visit alone. The surgery is filled with helpful staff, textbooks, diagnostic equipment and drugs. The visits case has an out-of-date bottle of penicillin, some blunt scissors and a packet of pills on which the label has faded, but they may be antibiotics, steroids, pain-killers or wormers. It is often hard to find the patient, let alone treat it efficiently. I once offered to visit an ailing koi carp, which had ulcers. When I arrived, the client took me down the garden and round a hedge, whereupon I was confronted by something which to my horrified gaze seemed rather like a sister to Lake Baikal. 'I think it's that one over there' the client said, helpfully pointing to a knot of fish about 15 feet from shore. I had to explain that without a sonar fish-finding device I was unlikely to be able to help on this occasion, and if he would like to somehow confine the fish I would return.

We should be aware that it is genuinely difficult for some clients to transport themselves or their pets to the clinic. Certain situations, such as euthanasia of old pets, may be more sympathetically dealt with in the home. Clients should be told of the reasons that the practice prefers not to visit unless necessary, and perhaps given suggestions as to alternative methods of getting the pet in. Friends and relatives may help, or have the number of a taxi firm which is happy to transport pets. If the client is still keen on a home visit, then they should be able to have one, unless it is unsafe for staff. Visits can be quite pleasant. They afford you a little time to think about the case as you drive there. You get to see inside a variety of homes. Tea and biscuits may be produced. On a more mercenary level, the taxman and your boss are unlikely to be persuaded that you need a car for work if no visits are carried out.

Explain to clients that there are times when it is more convenient for a vet to visit, and try to get them to give

for a living. Their awareness of the mysteries of circulation,
imination and respiration are cloudy to say the least.
u should be plain and simple in your explanations. It is better
ase of cystic calculi in elementary terms to a client who turns
rologist than to confuse the average layperson.

to get details of history and messages directly from clients
le. When a middle man is involved, information is often mud-
ves the 'benefit' of the messenger's interpretation. This may
misleading. Often what is passed on as an unhappy comment
t proves to be something completely different once you have
nity to get the facts directly from the owner concerned.
omments which you make may be taken the wrong way if
the client. Be cautious, accurate and discreet.

ent disagreements with colleagues

dividuals, and there is no reason why two veterinary surgeons,
he same practice, should have the same views on a case. On the
it gives the clients more confidence if the members of a prac-
sent a more or less uniform approach. No one is going to be
f they see a succession of vets who each have a different theo-
eir pet, and who change the patient's treatment at every visit.
hould see a case, therefore, where you find that you do disagree
inking that has gone before, tread carefully. Before changing the
f therapy, consult with the vet who has been dealing with the
e sure that the client knows that you are conferring. Any new
ld be presented as a joint effort to ensure that no criticism of the
owever slight, is implied. Confirm to the client the logic of the
vestigations and treatment, and give them sound reasons why it
idea to try something different.

y find on occasion that you will inadvertently contradict some-
another vet in the practice has said to a client. Few things are cut
in veterinary medicine, so point this out to the client. Accept the
s point of view and gently make the case for your own, while
hat there may be more than one way of thinking on the subject.

ebtors

ecome more experienced and confident in practice, you will
omewhat tougher in your approach towards bad debtors, I have

enough notice that a mutually acceptable time can be arranged. Get the lay staff to find out exactly what the visit is for, so that the visits case can be stocked up with the correct drugs and diagnostic equipment. If you are going to be delayed, ensure that the client is kept up to date with your progress. Explain to the client beforehand that most cases are going to need seeing on more than one occasion, so that they should take this into consideration when calculating whether they can afford a visit. Finally, if it really is too difficult at a certain time for a vet to go out to a patient, consider getting a member of the lay staff to collect the pet and return it to the clinic for treatment.

Mistakes

It really is best by dint of attention to detail, good communication with clients, lay staff and colleagues, and a good protocol for everyday situations, to avoid making mistakes. They will always happen on occasions, however. They may range from annoyances, such as forgetting to give the client some medication, or an error in the bill, or forgetting to order a special item in, to more serious errors with implications for the pet's health and treatment. It is best to be open, honest and apologetic about errors where possible. Offer to put things right as best you or your staff can and ascertain whether the client is happy with this. If they are not, discuss what would make them happy. It really is far better to accept a small loss in order to retain a happy client.

In more serious cases, you should be consulting your principal or partners for guidance. The matter may well be taken out of your hands. The vast majority of practices are very supportive of their assistants, and they will back you up and help you to sort out the problem to everyone's satisfaction, if possible. Let me again sound a note of caution if you feel that you have made a serious error. Don't admit anything to the client until your have obtained the guidance of your senior colleagues, and even your professional indemnity insurers. They will tell you what you may or may not do to deal with your client

Complaints

It is a fortunate vet, or a deaf one, who goes through his or her career without hearing a few complaints from clients. These may be justified or unjustified, but they will crop up.

Don't feel mortally offended if a client complains. We all have a right to complain if we feel we have not received the best service, and we are more likely to complain on behalf of our friends, children or pets than we are for ourselves. The stress of coping with a pet's illness can make clients unreasonable at times, and we should be aware of this at all times, not condemning them as miserable old so and so's because they have had the temerity to question us or our methods. We are not always right, and we don't always take the best course of action for pet or client, although this may not become apparent until we have the benefit of hindsight. Being prepared to listen to and investigate complaints will reduce the number of clients who simply leave for a second opinion without giving you a chance to explain yourself.

When a client complains, about you, a colleague or staff, take the time to listen to them. Ideally take them to a quiet room where you can discuss things with them and without the clients in the waiting room listening in. Allow the client to explain what it is that they are not happy with. It may be a case of misunderstanding, or it may be a genuine failing on the part of the practice. Be open minded. If you are able to explain the matter there and then, do so. If you would like to look into the circumstances and find out more facts, perhaps get someone else's point of view, or if you need to consult senior colleagues, explain this to the client. Promise to contact them by a certain time, and be sure to do so. Even if you are not able to give them the practice's final decision, call them to let them know that the matter is in hand, and make a new date to contact them. In either case you might be well advised to write a soothing letter, even if you have found that the practice has done nothing wrong.

It is well worth taking the time and trouble to deal with complaints fairly and pleasantly. For one thing each complaint can help the practice to be more client friendly. For another, a client who has a complaint well dealt with is actually likely to be an even better client afterwards, and to give you positive publicity.

Animals which won't get better

Some cases can be inordinately stubborn. Some are not going to get better because they are chronic conditions, and your treatment is simply going to be palliative. Skins, ears, gingivitis and endocrine disease come to mind, but there are many incidences. These diseases are going to test a client's patience to the limit because of the ongoing or recurring discomfort that the pet suffers, and the ongoing or recurrent hole that it puts in the bank account.

You've guessed it, I'm sure. Client communications are the answer.

When you see a case which is likely this at the outset. There are sever these conditions, with differing le options to the client. Our tendenc soften the blow of each visit for t opportunity to express an opinion prepared for you to carry out a thor early stage.

Keep owners well informed of th correspondingly get regular updates and response to treatment. Make e sees one vet most of the time, as it i deal with the patient for a consulta familiar with the whole case.

Be happy in your own mind that t nature of the complaint, and underst sultations with you. All too many ski short bursts of two or three consultati seeing different vets on each occasion of which may give temporary relief bu ment plan. Client education materia understanding. Many clients are not aw for example, has been diagnosed in thei long. When they see that a good impro assume that a cure has been achieved, an ment. Convince the client that you do k by keeping up to date with the latest t quite capable of absorbing news of rese

Rather than causing clients frustratio set. They should know how challenging what hard work they are causing you. G part of the team. Then they can share in and relapses.

Misunderstandings

Misunderstandings can be very annoying them by being clear in your record keepin and in your explanations to clients. Don't sion about medical matters in your clients average client has little idea of where the l

what it does digestion, e Therefore y to explain a out to be a u

It is best where possi dled or rece prove most from a clien the opportu Similarly, c passed on t

Inadver

We are all i even from other hand tice can pr impressed ry about th

If you s with the th direction case, and ideas shou first vet, h previous i may be an

You ma thing that and dried other vet allowing

Bad d

As you become

no doubt. As a younger vet, however, you may feel embarrassed about tackling debtors, insisting on payment or refusing them treatment for their pets. Debtors tend to come in two species. There are those who have genuinely been caught out, have had every intention of paying but have not been able to find the money. The other breed are the more habitual debtors, who are practised at failing to pay for services they receive, and not only from vets. Without wishing to generalise too much, these are individuals who can manage to find money for cigarettes, beer and mobile phones, but who don't wish to waste their money on paying you. These latter customers are past masters at appealing to your better nature, aiming to make you feel guilty for denying their pet treatment.

Firstly remember that you and the practice are perfectly entitled to expect payment for any services or drugs that you provide. Veterinary practices are not charities, and there are charities where genuinely needy clients can seek help. There is no reason why you should be made to feel guilty because someone who cannot afford the proper care that an animal requires, has decided to go out and buy or acquire a pet. It is a ludicrous situation to expect you to provide them with free or cheap treatment. Imagine the response if they went to their local garage and expected them to provide free servicing and repair for their car, as they had been able to buy one but not to keep it running. Because we are dealing with living creatures, we are subject to very effective emotional blackmail, but you are not responsible for the pet's problems.

The major problems arise when you are presented with a patient which needs therapy, but where you know that the owner is either unlikely to pay, or is a habitual debtor. The *Guide to Professional Conduct* states that

the practising veterinarian must ensure that any animal which may be suffering is seen irrespective of its owner's financial circumstances, to assess its need for immediate or emergency treatment and to relieve suffering without undue delay before it is referred to a colleague in an animal charity.

I have left the last part un-highlighted because many of us work in parts of the country where it isn't simply a question of sending the owner down the road to the nearest charity, as there isn't one within fifty miles. In truth almost all vets would automatically see an animal in need of treatment, but it is possible to provide relief from suffering quite cheaply either with low cost drugs or, if indicated, by euthanasia. You are not obliged to spend your practice's money on expensive treatment or investigation, and don't allow the owner to make you feel guilty about this. There is no Royal College of Television Repair Men with a corresponding clause in their guide to professional conduct, stating that 'it is the responsibility of all repair men to ensure that any TV set in need of urgent attention is repaired without delay in order to avoid undue suffering to its owners'.

Pets are a luxury, however soft we all are about them. If you are fortunate enough to work somewhere that benefits from charity clinics, you can refer the client on, after providing first aid. Those of us in less fortunate positions can seek help from charities in the way of funding, but they will not cover the whole cost of treatment, and if the debtor is a habitual offender it may be asking too much of your practice's good nature to face providing fifty per cent of the pet's treatment for free.

If you are aware that clients have had trouble paying your bills in the past, and I would recommend that the practice has a method of identifying those individuals, then be restrained in your approach to their pets' healthcare in the future. This is not only to avoid running up debts, but also to reduce the burden on a client who is likely to be struggling to make ends meet. After all, we don't want to give owners an excuse to ignore or neglect their pet's disorders, or to leave them until they require drastic measures to correct them. Try some of the following:

1) Although we enjoy providing high quality, logical and scientific veterinary medicine, is it strictly necessary in all cases? Do you really need confirmatory blood tests, or do you need to have culture results before treating an infection? Is that x-ray, ecg or ultrasound essential? Does the dog need a general anaesthetic to examine its ears before commencing treatment? Many older vets would say that we rely too heavily on laboratory and other tests, and we should exercise our diagnostic skills more. These are perhaps good cases to practise this philosophy on.

2) Modern drugs such as non-steroidal anti-inflammatories, antibiotics and flea treatments are wonderful. They provide a good range of treatment options with a high safety index. Are they really vital in all cases? Would an older pain killer costing a penny or two for a tablet be that much worse than the modern effective but expensive drugs? Isn't it better that the client uses a cheap anti-inflammatory in the long term, rather than one bottle of an expensive one which they won't repeat because of the cost? When treating heart disease, although ACE inhibitors are undoubtedly a fantastic advance in therapy, couldn't you improve the pet's quality of life with cheap drugs such as frusemide and digoxin? And if you wish to retain your boss's goodwill as well as the client's, please don't allow the client to walk out of the surgery with a 500ml bottle of fipronil for their pet's fleas allergy unless they pay at the time.

3) Good practice dictates that we see a patient, then have regular follow-up consultations until we are happy that the condition is resolved or controlled. This is laudable, but when dealing with a simple condition

for a less well off client, ask yourself if it is necessary to have them back in at all. If it is, can you get by with fewer visits at longer intervals? One incidence where you may positively want them to return regularly is the one where they haven't paid and you want to keep nagging them, but it does little good to keep building up the bill. Where the patients are on long-term therapy, increase the interval between regular checks to the maximum.

4) Some debtors are simply bad at managing their finances, and sudden expenses that crop up such as veterinary fees put too much strain on the available funds. Encourage these clients to budget for their pets. They may be able to afford £10 a month on an insurance policy, or they may be able to pay the money to your practice monthly as a budget account. Explain to clients that when they demonstrate commitment like this to meeting the costs of their pets' care, you in turn will be more willing to allow some credit when necessary.

Bad debtors are a feature of all businesses and all practices. To avoid them altogether is not an option. By being careful a practice can limit its losses to such debtors to an insignificant amount in terms of the value of materials given out. A sympathetic approach (NOT a soft approach) will encourage those clients who are not hardened debtors but genuinely needy to do all they can to provide for their pets' healthcare.

Shedding clients

There are clients who the practice may well be better off without. Habitual debtors, constant complainers (if unjustified), rude and unpleasant clients. Such clients do not add to the pleasure of being in practice, and most practices can well afford to shed them. It is not acceptable to do this too abruptly. When an unpopular client walks into your consulting room, that is not a good time to say 'I'm sorry Mrs Frogspawn, we don't like you so you'll have to go somewhere else'. You should not wait until a client has an urgent case to bring in, when you will be obliged to treat it and prolong your acquaintance.

This is not a decision to be taken lightly, and it is self-evident that it should only be taken with the backing and permission of the partners, who should proceed with the expulsion themselves. Some practices may be willing to accept any client as long as the colour of their money is good. When the decision has been made that the client has to go, a letter should be drawn up. Explain the problem as you see it: never paid a bill yet, rude to staff, always criticising staff and treatment, disruptive in the waiting room, unjustifiable complaints. Explain that the client's behaviour has led to a irretrievable breakdown in trust between vets and client, and that consequently it would seem difficult for that person to remain a client of the practice. Give them a period of notice, say 14 days, to find themselves a new practice, after which time they will not be seen as a client. If they would be good enough to inform you when they have chosen another practice, you will be delighted to send copies of the history to them. Sit back and give sigh of relief.

I have only had to sack a few clients, and in fact I am hard pressed to recall one who didn't in fact return to the practice, albeit in more subdued form. Remember that even though you have given notice to a client that they are no longer welcome, you may not refuse to examine their pet if is in urgent need of treatment. You may not need to give treatment, but if it is necessary then you are still obliged to do so, even if you know that you will not be paid. Hopefully, though, the situation won't arise once you have treated yourself to the ejection of a bad penny.

- Always be professional and respectful of colleagues when seeing second opinions
- Referring clients before they seek a second opinion will benefit both client and practice
- Don't be affronted if your client seeks a second opinion
- You should always have offered to see the patient if called out of hours
- Be very careful when accepting an owner's assessment of an out-of-hours case on the telephone
- Don't react negatively to complaints
- You are not always in the right, so don't dismiss complaints
- A helpful, fair response to complaints will enhance the practice's reputation
- Successful management of long-term cases relies on good communication with the client
- Avoid misunderstandings with clients or colleagues by attention to detail and communication
- Be firm when dealing with debtors: you are obliged to alleviate suffering, you are not obliged to throw good money after bad
- Practices should be prepared to shed genuinely unpleasant or disruptive clients

---

9

Euthanasia

O, let him pass. He hates him
That would upon the rack of this tough world
Stretch him out longer.

William Shakespeare, *King Lear*, V. iii.

Some years ago I wrote a book on the care of elderly dogs. It was packed, as I thought, with useful information on coping with a dog's advancing age, tips about making its life comfortable and details of the disorders of old age that one might be expected to come across. Whenever a client came up to me to say that they had read the book, however, all they ever seemed to mention was Chapter 11. 'Oh, it was so touching. It made me cry buckets.' 'It really brought things home to me.' 'I found it such a comfort.' You will have guessed I'm sure that Chapter 11 dealt with the thorny problem of death and euthanasia.

I'm afraid that this is something that you will find through your working career. You may be a brilliant practitioner, a skilled surgeon and a highly-motivated vet, but your clients will judge you not by your ability to preserve and prolong life, but by your proficiency at ending it. We receive far more cards, flowers and presents for putting pets to sleep than we ever do for piecing together broken limbs or staying up all night to unravel gastric torsions. This reflects the emotional nature of those final days and moments; the anguish that they cause clients. If we are able to help them through this difficult time gently and sympathetically, naturally they will remember this and be grateful.

The gift of euthanasia

Euthanasia comes from the Greek for 'a gentle death'. What a beautiful way to describe the process. This is what we should invariably be striving to achieve. Euthanasia is a very emotional procedure, for the veterinary surgeon as well as the client. In fact, the least concerned being present is usually the animal being despatched. I would hope that it remains an emotional process for most of us throughout our careers. When it becomes just another job and we become hardened to it, we lose a little of our humanity.

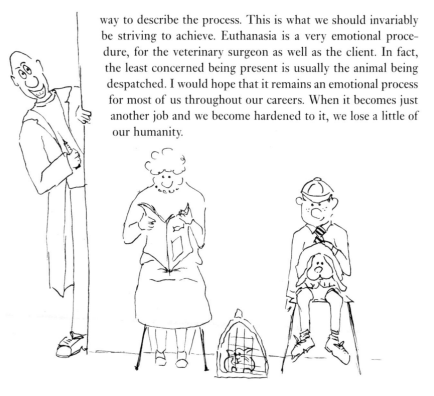

As sure as you won't go far in your career without someone mentioning St James Herriot, you will very soon be told by a client that they wish that euthanasia was available for humans. You will hear several gruesome ways to die experienced by relatives and friends of clients. You will also hear of obnoxious neighbours and various politicians whom clients would like to propose as candidates for euthanasia, but I suspect they are straying from the point.

It is true that we have a great gift in our hands. We are able to avoid suffering and to quickly and painlessly bring a life to an end. I think that in most cases there is no doubt that were the animal given a choice it would place its mark on the consent form. Far harder to deal with is the psychological strains that the decision to opt for euthanasia place upon our clients, both before and after the event. It will be hard on you in your first days in practice to be expected to be an emotional crutch for clients you don't know well, and who are much older than you. It is important to overcome your embarrassment and your own involvement so that you can support clients and guide them through this time. What a difficult tightrope we have to walk between remaining clinically detached, important if we are to provide the right advice, and allowing some emotion and sympathy to show through, which is vital to helping clients with their feelings and if we are to be more than glorified slaughtermen. Here as in no other area of your job you will need to use your psychiatric nursing skills. Clients react in many ways to losing their pets. They may be angry (at you or at themselves) or guilty, they may be weepy, brave, nonchalant, grateful, ungrateful, distraught to the point of collapse. They may bounce back quickly or be so upset that they will still be asking you if they have done the right thing in years to come. They may feel unable to keep another pet because they couldn't face losing one again.

You need to be able to sense the way in which an owner wants you to react or to help them. You have to discern whether you should be comforting them or whether they wish to be left alone with their feelings. Only practice and keen observation of your clients will help you to perfect your handling of clients in such trying times. To start with, don't become so wrapped up in your own feelings that you can seem distant and uncaring to the client. I know only too well that the responsibility of advising euthanasia, and the worry of performing the task well and efficiently, can preoccupy a young vet, but the client needs you more than the pet does at this time. Take the time to speak to them, ask them if they are all right and see if you can do anything to ease their distress.

Responsibilities

Euthanasia is a wonderful resource that we have in our armoury. It enables us to cut short suffering and pointless treatment. It spares a pet and its owner from the most unpleasant and upsetting segments of the course of a disease. It is one service which many doctors envy us the ability to provide. Doctors, however, are spared the soul searching which we have to go through when considering euthanasia. Sometimes it would be easier not to have the option, so that you knew what your course of action must be – to provide medical care to the bitter end. In almost all cases, however, it is preferable to help the patient on their way before they die of their illness.

There are times when euthanasia may seem too easy an option. If a client requests euthanasia even though in your opinion the condition is eminently treatable, what do you do? Clients may request this because they think that they may be sparing the pet suffering, because they can't face the emotional trauma of treatment, because they can't afford prolonged treatment, because they are due to go on holiday or because Christmas is coming and they don't want an incontinent dog soiling the carpet in front of the relatives. There are all too many reasons for requesting euthanasia.

Should euthanasia simply be the easy option? Can you refuse to perform euthanasia if that is the client's wish? Strictly speaking, you are not under an obligation to perform treatment, including euthanasia, simply because an owner tells you to perform it, unless by not carrying out the treatment the animal will be subject to unnecessary suffering. Therefore if euthanasia is not necessary, you do not have to perform it at the owner's request. Will it benefit the animal if you don't, though? If the owner has lost the will to continue caring for the pet, might not the pet's best interests be served by euthanasia? Here are points for many hours of discussion. You may ask the owner to sign the pet over to you for treatment and re-homing (and be sure that you do get written agreement) but a practice can accumulate many unwanted animals in this way. Never agree to put a pet to sleep and then surreptitiously find it a home. If the situation arises we ask the owner to sign for permission to re-home if possible, and for euthanasia if we should be unable to find a home.

You in turn need to examine your motives when recommending euthanasia. Do you truly have the animal's best interests at heart? Are you advising cutting short the pet's life because you feel that it cannot comfortably continue, or because further treatment is going to be difficult and unrewarding? Are you merely trying to avoid a complicated and time-consuming piece of surgery with involved aftercare? Is euthanasia a quick answer when you think the owner might be disturbing you too much over the course of the next few days (and nights)? You may not even realise that these considerations are passing through your mind. The subconscious is very powerful. You have in your control something which few other people truly possess: the power of life or death over another living creature. A creature, moreover, which in many people's eyes is an important part of their family. Never become hardened or immune to the truth of what you are doing – taking away the gift of life.

The veiled request for euthanasia

Some clients will do all that they can to avoid actually asking for euthanasia. They may feel guilty about doing so, or be too embarrassed to ask. You need to develop your ability to identify the veiled request for euthanasia. It is important to detect it, because these clients will go so far as to allow you to carry out lengthy and expensive treatment on their pets simply because they cannot bring themselves to speak their mind. You may find that you have performed wonders to pull an 18-year-old cat through a bout of acute kidney failure, and yet receive no thanks for doing so, because in their heart of hearts the clients had felt that enough was enough and the cat wouldn't live long enough to justify all the attention. You may even find yourself the subject of bitter complaints if, for example, you try heroically to operate on an old dog with an intestinal tumour, only for it to die a few days after surgery. 'All we wanted was to put the dog out of its suffering', the clients will claim, even though they never thought to mention this.

In cases where euthanasia might be considered an option, however unlikely, do at least discuss the possibility with the clients. You should be presenting them with treatment options and this is after all one of them, particularly in elderly animals. They may leap at the offer. They may be horrified that you are considering it, but you should be able to discuss it in a way which doesn't offend most clients.

Watch for clients who repeatedly comment on the age of a pet, or the fact that they don't want it to suffer. They have often made up their minds before coming to see you that what they would like is euthanasia, but for the sake of their consciences they would like you to be the one to mention it first. Don't try too hard to persuade these clients that the pet is quite capable of coming through the illness that it is suffering. If you are wrong and the pet succumbs or has to be put down a few days later, you are the bad guy, only interested in making a buck or two, never mind the pet's welfare. If you are successful in your treatment, the clients are stuck with an elderly pet which they had decided to let go.

You may well disagree with the client's decision in such cases, but please refrain from being churlish or trying to make the client feel guilty. Even if you cannot entirely understand their desire for euthanasia, that doesn't mean that they love their pet any the less. They feel that they are making the best choice for their pet. You should ensure that you are sympathetic and even if you can't bring yourself to say that they have done the right thing, never make them feel that they have done the wrong thing.

Persuading a client

Some clients are so loathe to lose their pets that they will drag things out to the bitter end. They are prepared to put up with all manner of inconvenience themselves in order to keep the animal alive as long as possible. In the main, these owners have lost sight of what is best for the pet, and are simply continuing for their own sakes. They will often recognise this after the pet has died, but they may be mortally offended if you were to suggest that they were being selfish while the pet still draws breath. They may not see the suffering of the animal, deluding themselves that the odd wag of a tail or purr is a sign that the pet is still enjoying life.

These are delicate cases to deal with. As a matter of principle, it should always be the client's decision to opt for euthanasia. You may advise and recommend, but you should not force the issue or insist. Clients will ask you to decide for them, but you must gently inform them that the decision is theirs alone. In practice it may well be you who is deciding that enough is enough, but you must be instructed by the client before you can go ahead.

To begin with, don't hide from a client the discomfort and distress that a pet may be going through, just to spare their feelings. Be honest. The client is rarely able to assess whether their pet is truly comfortable. These are people who will place a cat which has been hit by a car on your table, two legs and a jaw broken and the left eye prolapsed, and say 'Well at least it can't be in pain because it's still purring'. They will tell you that they know their dog is happy because it is still eating. For goodness sakes, some Labradors will still eat six months after they have died and been cremated. You are in the position to draw this to the owner's attention, but gently. Owners are not cruel, just a little blind to the facts at times.

You will be asked what you 'honestly think' about cases. Be honest. If you think that the prospects are poor or that there is no way to alleviate discomfort, say so. You will be asked if you think 'that I'm doing the right thing?' Point out that the condition of the pet and past experience with similar cases means that there is little prospect of improvement, and that 'we' are probably just delaying the inevitable. The use of 'we' when discussing cases will give the client some moral support in their decision, without taking away that decision from them. They will ask you what you would do if the pet were yours, and again you should be honest, or even a little dishonest if it helps to bring about the correct decision for the pet.

We should all sympathise with these clients, and not condemn them for their inability to make the right decision early enough. We all hope that when the time comes for us to decide upon our own pets' future we will be strong enough to do the right thing.

Recognising the 'right time'

Clients often worry that they won't in fact be able to decide when the right time is to let their pets go. They will ask you for guidance, looking for pointers that will tell them that the time has come. These are clients who recognise that they may hang on too long for selfish reasons. It may sound trite, but my usual advice to these people is that they will know when the time is right. To me, the fact that they have had the foresight to think about this early on shows that they are to some extent aware of the balance between keeping a pet for as long as possible and allowing it to depart this earth with some dignity. Many of these clients have said to me afterwards that they did indeed sense when the appropriate time had arrived.

You can help with some pointers. For most dogs, enjoyment of life involves exercise, food and the company of their owners. If they are no longer able to exercise, they may still be content if they have contact with their owner and are able to feed. Once they lose interest in food, or feeding is difficult, or when they are only vaguely aware of their owners, it is probably time to say goodbye. A pet is entitled to be comfortable. If they are afflicted by a chronic condition which is painful, once the drugs they are receiving fail to adequately control discomfort, the pet should be allowed to go. If a pet requires a level of attention which the owner is, with the best will in the world, unable to provide, then the pet should go. Incontinence, both faecal and urinary, is not just unpleasant for the owner. It causes most pets distress, and is unhygienic. If uncontrollable they are grounds for euthanasia. While considering what is fair for the pet, don't forget the owner. If keeping the pet alive is causing anguish for the client, they should be gently steered towards euthanasia. They may well delay, feeling that they are letting the pet down by giving up on them, until they become ill themselves. Remember that pets, especially dogs, are extremely sensitive to the state of mind of their owners. If the owner is permanently upset, the pet is likely to be in a constant state of stress as well.

Where to do the deed

There is a certain natural reluctance for small animal vets to leave the surgery premises if they can help it. There are many logical arguments in favour of performing euthanasia at the surgery. The procedure can be carried out efficiently with plenty of help available. The body can be quickly and discreetly moved for disposal. It takes up far less of the vet's time. The vet, being in her home environment, feels more relaxed and confident, and can therefore do a better job. You may want to relay some, but not all of these arguments to the client.

Many owners, on the other hand, nourish a desire to have their pet's final moments at home. They would rather that the pet is in familiar surroundings, not stressed by being brought to the surgery where it may have had some unpleasant experiences, and will certainly not be so relaxed. The owners too may feel that to be at the surgery at such a time may be too upsetting for them. They may feel that they will be embarrassed when they inevitably give way to their emotions in front of strangers.

There are certainly pros and cons for both options. I feel that we should at least be prepared to comply with the owners' wishes as long as they are fully aware of what will be involved. It is hard, for instance, to spirit away a body from someone's house, especially if the body happens to belong to a bull mastiff. They will have to see you wrap the body and carry it to the car, and then lay it in the boot. This in itself may prove very upsetting. Are they ready for this? There is naturally a cost consideration to be taken into account.

Dogs may be turn out to be either easier or harder to deal with in their home environment. They will feel more confident, and in a dog with aggressive tendencies this may be a problem. Many dogs are aggressive at the surgery through nervousness and fear, and they may well be more tolerant at home. You can always use as high a dose of tranquillizers as you wish, one of the compensations of having to perform such a terminal task.

If you are to visit a pet for euthanasia, ask the owners to give you as much notice as possible. Preferably the appointment should be booked some days in advance. They should be able to arrange a time which is convenient for you, when you and probably a nurse can reasonably leave the surgery. The pet should be of a temperament which will ensure that the procedure is calm and safe for all concerned. The method of disposal of the carcass should have been decided in advance.

Euthanasia can be performed in a very peaceful way in the home, which will be of great comfort to the client, leaving them without any sense of regret or undue distress. An old pet may be helped on its way while lying in its bed, almost unaware that anything untoward is happening. If it is within your power, and bearing in mind that in many areas and situations it is not practical, should you deny that opportunity to your client and patient?

When to do the deed

Be sensitive to your clients' feelings when scheduling appointments for euthanasia. You do not want to find that there is a pet to put down in the middle of a consulting period. Not only will you be pressurised and unable to devote the time that the clients and their pet deserve, but they will be forced to wait amidst other clients who have healthy pets, further upsetting the owner of the unfortunate animal whose time has come. When you have performed the task, the clients will have to depart through a busy waiting room, exposing their emotions for all to see. You will have a corpse to try to remove quickly, discreetly and respectfully. If you weren't behind before you started, you will be when you finish. Not only does it take a little time to carry out euthanasia gently, but the owners may well be unable to tear themselves away from their pet, or they may agonise for long minutes on whether they are making the correct decision before they allow you to administer the lethal injection. It is hard to be properly sympathetic when you have a queue of restless clients outside. The pressure of time will colour your judgement when you are advising the clients on whether it is actually the right course of action.

Ensure that lay staff are trained to offer appointments either outside of normal consulting hours, or at the ends of surgeries, so that you are not being rushed, and you can allow clients as long as they wish to be with their pet both before and after the event. Ideally use a spare room which is a little quieter than the rest, where you will be undisturbed. If there is a back entrance to the building which the clients can use, so much the better. Losing a much loved pet is going to be traumatic whatever we do, but we should strive to allow pets a quiet, peaceful and dignified exit for their sakes and the sakes of their owners.

How to do the deed

I may seem to be going beyond my brief in trying to advise on the actual act of euthanasia, but here is an area where a very bad impression may be given to clients. They do not always know what to expect if they have not experienced losing a pet in this way before. They will not be impressed if they see their pet handled roughly, hear it crying (in distress, as they think), see it struggling, see the vet vainly trying to find a vein, working from one leg to the other, or see the animal coming back to life after the vet has turned away with a sigh of relief. I know, and you will know, that any of these things can happen to any vet, however experienced and well prepared he might be. They are to us, used to seeing many deaths and many different reactions from the animals, unfortunate but normal possibilities. To the client, where this may be their only experience of euthanasia, they can be horrific and devastating. Imagine how they will describe a poor euthanasia to their friends. To them the vet will have been cruel, inefficient, incompetent. The pet was distressed, tortured, in pain. Few things can put a client off a vet like a bad euthanasia. Your aim should be firstly to avoid these distressing occurrences, and secondly to educate your clients so that they don't misinterpret quite normal happenings.

Before delivering an injection of pentobarbitone, find out whether the owners wish to be with their pet. Many would rather not be present at the last. It is debatable whether or not they should be present. From the pet's point of view, it is probably comforting to have a familiar smell and sound close at hand. If the owner is getting upset, even hysterical, then the pet will naturally become distressed where it may not have suspected anything untoward. If the owners decide to stay with their pet, see if they have had a pet put down before. If not, explain the process. Explain what you will do, that the pet will need to be restrained, how quickly the drug will cause them to succumb (hopefully), that some trembling and gasping after the event are quite normal and not signs of life, that the pet may open its bowels or urinate, and that animals will die with their eyes open. It is an unfortunate truth that the animals which are easiest to find a vein in and those which will drop dead most rapidly are young healthy pets with a good circulation. The older and more decrepit a pet is, the harder it will be to inject and the longer it will take for the drug to find its way to the brain. Explain this to the owner. Tell them that the pet might express displeasure, but that this is usually because they don't want to be restrained, and not because they are being hurt by either the intravenous injection, or the barbiturate entering its bloodstream. If they are taking their pet home for burial, do warn them that the pet may gasp even some time after death, or make a noise as they move it from the car.

Take whatever precautions you need to in order to ensure a smooth process. If a pet is fractious or nervous and likely to play up, use a heavy sedative beforehand. You may even use anaesthetic dosages quite happily. This is to be strongly recommended if you are single-handed at night at the surgery, or when you are visiting a client to perform euthanasia. I find it very useful to sedate cats heavily, enabling me to administer the final injection when the cat is lying peacefully in its bed or on the owner's lap. Acepromazine and ketamine work well together, administered subcutaneously for comfort. This combination avoids the retching and vomiting which may be seen with medetomidine and ketamine, and which the owner may interpret as distress in the pet. Be sure to have as much help as you need to do the job efficiently. Shave a large area so as to ensure that you hit the vein first time. Work in good light conditions. When on a visit, the client will often show you into a dimly lit corridor or pantry where the pet happens to be lying peacefully, but unless you can work out a method of I V by Braille, move the animal to a more suitable location. Wait until you are confident that you are securely in the vein before pressing the plunger. It is very upsetting for all concerned if the vein blows after you have only administered a fraction of the dose. You are then faced with trying to find another vein while the pet is in a state of semi-anaesthetised excitement, not only thrashing around but howling in a manner calculated to quail the staunchest client. If you are injecting a dog which is known to be untrustworthy, as well as sedating it, use a muzzle. The owner should appreciate that the safety of all is of paramount importance, and you can hardly be expected to do a good job if you are in fear of losing a finger or two. Once well in the vein, deliver the drug smoothly and steadily. Have one or more extra syringes already loaded, so that you can top up if necessary without an awkward pause while you hold on to the pet grimly and the nurse fumbles to reload another.

Be calm and authoritative. Don't allow the owner to upset the pet unduly. Of course they may wish to show their emotions, but there is little point in letting the pet know that this isn't just another blood sample or anaesthetic. Ask them to be reassuring to the pet, talking to it and stroking it. Talk to the pet yourself, in as soothing a manner as you can. This will calm the pet, the owner and yourself.

Consider the use of a saphenous vein in dogs, especially large dogs at home. It is often quite easy to access this vein while a dog is lying in its bed, thus allowing the owners to hold the dog's front end without interference. Dogs often object less to this vein being used compared to the cephalic in my experience.

Exotic pets

Furries, scalies and featheries often get a bit of a raw deal when it comes to euthanasia. Rather than a gentle intravenous injection and a swift death, they are sometimes subjected to vague proddings in the direction of the heart, and may slip away rather more slowly that their larger counterparts. An alternative is the 'gas chamber', with a chloroform-soaked piece of cotton wool in a tin or plastic container. This may be quite humane, but the pets seem to struggle a bit more than I find comfortable.

Rabbits and birds have perfectly accessible veins which afford a vet good practice on their IV technique while bringing a swift unconsciousness. Birds can be rapidly rendered unconscious with a small dose of isoflurane, allowing even easier access to the vein. This anaesthetic is also excellent for rapidly knocking down small mammals and reptiles before administering the *coup de grâce*. If owners wish to stay with their guinea pigs, hamsters or other small mammals at euthanasia, one of the injectable anaesthetic combinations is very useful.

Don't assume that owners these days are going to be any less upset about the loss of their rabbit or guinea pig than they are about losing a dog or cat. You will need to show that you can perform euthanasia just as humanely for these creatures as for your larger patients.

After the event

Having successfully despatched a pet, you must deal with the body and with the clients. Ask the clients if they would like to stay with the body for a few moments, on their own, to say their goodbyes. Don't rush them. You should have discussed the arrangements for disposal of the carcass before carrying out euthanasia. This is a poor time to ask them if they want the normal cremation service or to have the ashes returned. Urn, casket or box? Owners are unlikely to make an entirely rational decision at this moment.

A rather distasteful part of the proceedings is the question of payment. Give the client an opportunity to pay before seeing you, so as not to be bothered with paying afterwards. The vision of a client trying to hold back tears while waiting to pay at reception, the receptionist fumbling with the credit card machine, the till ringing – these are not pleasing images. Many practices feel that it is important to obtain payment for euthanasia at the time, as there is little incentive for clients to pay up once they have no pet to seek treatment for. I have some sympathy for this, but for established clients I am only too happy to offer to send a bill in the post, which gives an opportunity to send a note of condolence.

If the body has to be moved from a part of the practice where the public may see you, I would advise using a large blanket to wrap it up for transport. It is an unfortunate fact that most of our body bags are made from thick black plastic, and to the average client this equates to a bin bag. This seems to be an image that sticks firmly in the mind of the Joe public. It may be inevitable that the pet will end up in a black bag, but try to shield this from your clients. When visiting a home to carry out euthanasia, again take a suitable wrapping to transport the body from the house to your car. Far more pleasant for the client to see you use a shroud of some sort rather than folding the pet into a bag on the living room floor. Consider taking some form of stretcher if the pet is a large one so that you can move it from the house with some dignity.

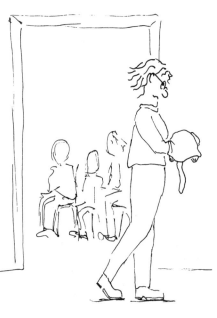

At all times show respect for the client and the pet's body, and ensure that your lay staff do likewise.

Disposal

In truth, once the spirit has departed, the body of a pet is no more than an inanimate object. The pet which the client has been so emotionally attached to is no longer there. Nevertheless there is an understandable wish to see that a pet's body is handled and disposed of with dignity. Here is an area where veterinary surgeons must exercise a great deal of tact.

The facts are that there is little alternative to packaging a body in some form of sealed plastic container and storing it in a freezer or cool room until the agency responsible for disposal arrives to collect it. They must then transport the body in the company of several other carcasses back to their premises where they will be burnt. I would hope that all clinics now use pet cremation services, thus satisfying health and safety regulations, waste disposal regulations and ensuring that pets receive as dignified an end as possible.

These raw facts may prove a little unpalatable for clients, used to the paraphernalia of human undertakers and funerals. The only ways for people to afford their pets this type of send-off are to have them at home for burial, with all the attendant problems, or to use a pet cemetery, which will often carry out a small 'service' and interment, at a cost. Individual cremation with or without the return of ashes is another possibility, at a premium. More and more clients are opting for the return of their ashes, and it is worth using a cremation service which can do this in a professional and sympathetic way, with a good quality casket or urn to hold the ashes and some way of reassuring the owner that it is in fact their pet which has been returned to them. A lock of hair in a card with the ashes is one method. A reputable agent will be happy for clients to visit or to take their own pets to the crematorium.

According to the letter of the law (The Environmental Protection Act 1990), it is not legal for owners to transport their dead pets from the practice back home for burial, since once they are dead, they are considered clinical waste, and only an authorised person may transport clinical waste. The BVA was assured by the Environment Minister that the law need not be interpreted in such a strict manner. If only all laws were so flexible.

We should do all we can to ensure that the bodies of our patients are treated with respect by all staff. Covering bodies with a blanket in the consulting room rather than placing them directly into a body bag will avoid offending clients' sensitivities. If the body has to be carried in view of the public, be sure to have enough people to do the job gently, without the carcass slipping or dropping, or with the carrier puffing and blowing. Use a stretcher if needs be. Carry small bodies cradled in your arms, not hanging down. Wrap bodies of small pets which are to be returned home in a towel you don't need or some clean paper. Even when out of sight of the public, please remain respectful of dead bodies and allow them some dignity. They may be no more than so much bone and flesh, but treating them with due regard pays some homage to their memory.

Planning ahead

The moments leading up to, during and following euthanasia are highly emotionally charged for client and vet alike. The stress and embarrassment may lead clients to make decisions, or fail to make decisions, that they may regret later. Somewhat like childbirth, the pain of the moment renders the afflicted irrational and vulnerable, so that it is better to have a birth (or a death) plan worked out when the mind is not rendered as useless as a jellyfish by current events.

Many people now plan for their own deaths in the most sensible and practical fashion. They pay for a funeral, choose the coffin, the method of disposal and the hymns to be sung. When the time comes for them to shuffle off their mortal coil, their loved ones are free to grieve and argue over the will without having to bother with the technicalities. You should encourage your clients to have a plan of action for the time when they must lose their pet. The following are the sort of decisions they might like to think over.

When and why

It is an idea to discuss with clients the circumstances which would decide them that the time had come for euthanasia. When they are able to consider it dispassionately, they may feel that there are certain pointers which they would consider reasons to let a pet go. It may be that the pet can't exercise much, is being sick daily, has lost too much weight, is having to have too high a dose of anti-inflammatories, needs a general anaesthetic at a stage when the owners don't think it would be fair, or one of a dozen other factors. If they haven't considered this beforehand, then they may be swayed at the time by either an overwhelming desire not to lose the pet, or by not wishing to give the impression that they don't care enough to continue treatment. They can always change their mind later on should they so desire. On a more practical level, nearer the time they can decide what time of day will be suitable for them, and when they can be attended by the vet that they usually see.

Where

It is much easier for the practice if a client can decide early on whether they wish for euthanasia at the surgery or at home, and perhaps whether or not they wish to be present. By not leaving it until there is a desperate need for euthanasia, the client can ensure that a vet is actually going to be free to come out. If they have chosen to come to the surgery they can choose a quiet time.

Disposal

These days a growing number of clients like the idea of having their pet's ashes returned. This is partly so that they will know where the ashes' final resting place is, and partly because they appreciate the more individual attention that their pet's body will receive. The problem is that this service is quite naturally considerably more expensive than a normal cremation. The vet may well feel too awkward about discussing such a financial outlay with a distraught owner. If the question is asked, the client may choose individual cremation when caught up by the emotion of the moment, and may regret it later. If individual cremation isn't suggested, the client may discover later that he could have chosen this option, but that it is by then too late. Far better to let the client know that such a service exists well in advance of the dreadful day, allowing them to make up their minds coolly and reasonably, and perhaps to save towards the cost. Should the client wish to bury a pet at home, you might point out that digging a hole three feet deep and large enough for a Labrador or German Shepherd dog is not the work of a moment. Far better to have the grave prepared in advance so as to lessen the upset of the moment.

Payment

The last thing you or your client really wants to intrude on their pet's final minutes is the mundane question of payment. If they know that the fateful day is approaching, they might like to consider pre-paying so that they don't need to deal with payment on the day. This will save you an unpleasant task as well.

The follow up

The last thing that you want a client to think is that once a pet is dead and gone you forget about them and their owners and move on to other patients which move about a bit more. Not only does this give a poor impression, but it is also usually very untrue. Vets become very fond of their patients and their clients. Very often they have worked hard to treat elderly patients and keep them healthy. Young animals which are terminally ill demand a great deal of medical and emotional input. It is sensible to communicate to owners that you are still thinking of them after they have lost their pet.

It is possible to buy pre-printed condolence cards now to be sent out automatically after the death of a pet. My feeling is that if you are going to make the effort to contact owners then you should be sincere, and be seen to be sincere. Sending out an impersonal communication simply reeks of wanting to be seen to be caring without actually being concerned, except with retaining the client's business. Consequently I would advise a hand-written letter, or sending a blank card with your communication inside.

When writing to an owner you should be expressing your condolences, reviewing the case, reassuring the owner that they have made the right decision in having their pet destroyed (if they haven't died) and trying to provide some consolation for the owner.

Owners are often affected by guilt and doubts after euthanasia. They may also not have fully understood the condition that their pet was affected by. Setting down on paper exactly what was wrong, and emphasising the aspects which would have caused enough distress to warrant euthanasia, will help them to accept the decision. Clients really want someone to say that they have done the right thing, and you should be able to give them this comfort, even if you haven't completely agreed with the decision or the timing. Point out the kindness they have done by allowing their pet to slip away peacefully rather than having to experience the latter stages of a terminal disease. If the pet has died, you may want to reassure the owners that they have done nothing wrong, that all that could have been done for the pet was done, and that it was peaceful and comfortable when it died.

Mention some characteristics or incidents which you recall about their pet to show that it was an individual to you, and not just one of the crowd. You may have known the pet for some time, and may be able to go over something from its early history. Perhaps the owners came by the pet in unusual circumstances or it was quite striking as a young animal. In most cases, a pet's illness only affects it for a relatively short period of its life, and you could suggest to owners that they try to remember the pet as it was in its prime, rather than during its final weeks or days.

Sadly, all animals will die. Their life spans in most cases being much shorter than our own, a pet owner is going to experience a few deaths if they wish to carry on owning pets. Although losing a pet can be devastating, this only reflects the level of pleasure that it gave to its owner while alive. Thus I don't feel that the upset caused by losing a pet is reason for not owning one. You will find yourself writing quite a number of letters of condolence. Inevitably you are going to find yourself repeating phrases, sentences and even whole letters. This is not important. What is important is that you are sincere and sympathetic in what you write. This, as much as anything else you do to care for your clients throughout their pet's life, will endear you to them and make them choose you to care for their next little bundle of joy.

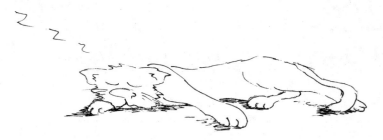

- Euthanasia is the procedure most likely to enhance (or detract from) your reputation
- Every client should receive sympathetic handling at this time
- Learn to recognise a request for euthanasia even when the clients can't bring themselves to spell it out
- You can advise and guide, but the client must be the one to decide on euthanasia
- Be sympathetic to owners' wishes about where euthanasia is performed
- Don't make owners feel rushed – schedule euthanasia for quiet periods
- Develop an efficient, smooth technique
- Treat carcasses with respect
- Death is inevitable – encourage owners to plan ahead
- Send letters of condolence, but be sincere

10

How to be a helpful client

Some characteristics of clients are so common, so consistently repeated, that there has long been a rumour that a manual of client behaviour exists. This document aims to guide clients on how to get the best from their veterinary surgery, how to be helpful and give the vet a more fulfilled life and some tips on money saving. A version of the guide was published some years ago, but few vets were able to see it. I have managed to get sight of a bootleg copy, and here reproduce some of the salient points.

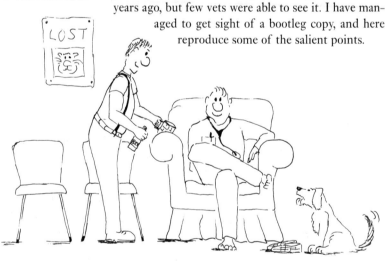

Top secret: How to have a happy vet

Appointments

Waste of time. Many surgeries now try to force you to make appointments. The problem is that this uses up staff time on the telephone, when they could be doing something useful, like seeing you. Appointments always tend to be at those awkward times, when you don't really want to come. When you have an appointment, you will probably also have to wait amongst several other clients, with their ill pets spreading nasty germs, and their owners very likely doing the same. Far better just to turn up unannounced, preferably outside of consulting hours. This will ensure that you are seen on your own with no distractions for the poor vet. Who wants a queue of clients waiting outside? One o'clock or just before is a good time – you might catch the vet as he is on his way out, with nothing else to do. The receptionist may be a little terse with you, but it's just a sign of affection.

If you have been silly enough to make an appointment, you might find that the vet is a few minutes late in seeing you. This means that some other client has pinched some time. Once you get into the consulting room, you must be sure to get your money's worth. Think up as many questions as you can to keep the vet's attention. If you run out of queries about the pet you have brought, ask about one you have left at home, or perhaps your mother's pet or a friend's.

■ **Top tip:** If you can wait until your pet looks really ill, you are likely to be seen immediately, whatever the time.

Not wasting the vet's time

Vets are busy people. Besides which they do cost a lot. Try to save their time and your money by getting some advice about your pet before taking it to the clinic. Suitable experts are the pet shop, the breeder, the groomer or the television. Vets really appreciate it if you can look up a disease on the internet, as they rarely have time to do this. Go in with a sheaf of papers on the disease which your pet has. You may even be able to tell your vet exactly what is wrong and what treatment should be prescribed.

Vets are well known to have a fascination with body waste. They very much appreciate a chance to examine your pet's emissions. Never visit without taking a sample of vomit or diarrhoea, the slimier and smellier the better. Try to collect it in some absorbent paper which will become nicely saturated with the sample, enabling the vet to feel the texture of the excretion as she unwraps it.

You will usually be asked to return to the surgery to check your pet's response to treatment. This wastes everybody's time. Pets always get better, so don't bother returning. Just go back once a month when the symptoms recur.

Hold on to any medication that you have left over once your pet recovers. You can ensure that you have some left by not using the whole of the course of treatment you have been given. You will always be given too much anyway. When your pet is next ill, work your way through the tablets, ear and eye drops and potions that you have in your medicine chest. Don't worry about the 'Use by' dates – they are just put there to satisfy EU bureaucrats. The vet will appreciate your efforts to save her time.

- **Top tip:** Get a friend to keep their excess medication as well. This doubles your chances of finding something to treat your pet with.

Control of your pet

The vet loves to see a well-trained animal. When you enter the consulting room with your dog, pat the table and give the command 'Up'. Funnily enough, your dog probably won't obey you. Can't imagine why not. Other useful commands to try out are 'sit' and 'down'. It's possibly because your dog is so excited to see her favourite vet, but she probably won't perform these tricks either, but you should show the vet that you know what they mean.

If you are taking a cat in, place the carrier on the table, open the door and tell the cat firmly to come out. You'll be amazed how often it doesn't actually do this. Fortunately vets enjoy thrusting their arms deep into cat carriers to extract cats. You can make this a little more fun by buying the longest carrier with the narrowest opening, and by providing plenty of blankets for the cat to hide under. Another method of entertainment if you have a wicker basket is to lose the original straps, and tie the basket up with string. A couple of really tight granny knots make for minutes of diversion.

Nothing impresses more than a well-trained bird. Let your budgie or parrot out of its cage quickly, before the vet can stop you, then as it flies around the room, try holding a finger out and calling it to land. The bird probably won't respond, but vets do like stalking birds with a towel which they throw over the creatures with great panache.

- **Top tip:** See if you can train your dog to leap up at the vet, which shows great affection for the 'doctor'. If you can walk the dog through a muddy field beforehand, the vet will be able to show the stains to other clients, thus showing how much her patients love her.

Dangerous pets

Everyone knows that the most important factor when dealing with an unfriendly creature is to have confidence. It is important for your vet's welfare that you don't warn him if your pet tends to be a bit cranky. Let him deal with him as though he was just a cuddly bundle of fluff, and hopefully no one will get hurt. Once the vet has got to grips with your pet, it is quite permissible to let him know that he is doing very well. For instance, if your vet has prised open your Rottweiler's mouth and is closely examining its throat, encourage him by declaring 'Well! He's never let anyone do *that* before!' If your cat has just caused the vet to back off while sucking a bitten thumb, console him by telling him 'He must like you. He sat on the last vet's head and scratched his wig off.' And don't forget that every vet loves to be reassured when he opens your hamster's cage: 'Don't worry, he's never bitten anyone before.'

■ **Top tip:** Never tell your pet off when it has injured the vet. It needs calming and reassurance, so tell it what a good boy it has been and give it a treat.

Handling pets

Vets don't like you to hold on to your animals too tightly. It restricts the pet's movements and so masks symptoms from the vet. If the vet is looking in an ear or clipping claws, for instance, just hold the pet's head lightly. If it tries to bite the vet, that gives him valuable information; in this case, that something hurts.

If the vet wants to examine some anal glands or take a temperature, tell your dog to sit. This is very helpful. If your pet is having a blood sample taken, with a nurse holding it, talk to the pet just as the vet inserts the needle. Your pet needs distraction and reassurance at this time. Don't worry if it struggles a bit – it just wants to come and see you.

Try allowing your parrot or cat to sit on your shoulder while the vet has a look at it. This allows the vet a good upward view at the animal – especially helpful if the vet is 5'2" and you are 6'5". This has the added advantage of giving the pet confidence in a stressful situation.

■ **Top tip:** Should you be asked to put a muzzle on your dog, be sure not to do it up too tight, or even at all tightly. This way the dog can always get out of it should there be an emergency.

Children

Yes please! A vital accessory for the client. Vets love children and the more the merrier. At least two are required. If you don't have enough children of your own, you can always borrow some. Grandchildren, nephews and nieces, the neighbour's children or a rota from the local primary school – any source will do. It's so good for children to see what goes on at the vet's. They have a unique opportunity to handle all sorts of delicate equipment, and may even learn that needles are sharp and best poked in other children. It's so refreshing to visit a place where you don't need to keep the little poppets under close control. If they are being a nuisance the vet will surely tell you so.

- **Top tip:** Encourage children to speak to the vet and offer their stuffed toys for treatment, but *don't* let them tell the vet the truth about how long the pet has really been ill, or how many doses of medication you have missed.

Answering questions

Vets find it very boring if you actually answer the question that they have asked you. Remember, these are intelligent people, and it is an insult to them to think that they are not capable of deducing the correct reply. To spice up consultations for them, be just a little evasive when questioned. Some examples might be:

Vet: 'How old is Roger?'
Client: 'Well, we got him when we moved house, didn't we Norman?'

V: 'How many times has Icky been sick?'
C: 'Oh, all night.'

V: 'How long has Twiggy been off her food?'
C: 'Well, she's never really eaten since we got her.'

V: 'Is Fester vaccinated?'
C: 'Oh yes. He had all his jabs when he was a kitten.'
V: 'And how old is he now?'
C: 'Well, we got him when our Shareen was born. Oh, sorry. That was just 16 years ago.'

It is best to hide the odd bit of information from the vet. For instance, if your Jack Russell terrier has a touch of the runs and you tell the vet that you shared last night's rat vindaloo with him, she will put the diarrhoea down to this and possibly miss some serious disorder. Just tell her the bare minimum.

- **Top tip:** Everyone likes a double act, so take your spouse along to help with entertaining the vet. Be sure to get your stories straight before you see the vet. Whatever you do, you don't want to inadvertently agree with each other.

Listening to the vet

Don't waste time at the surgery listening to what the vet has to say. There are far too many other things to grab your attention. Look at the useful and pretty posters on the consulting room walls. See what new instruments have been added since your last visit. Is the new ophthalmoscope better than the one your son broke last time? Can you read anything of interest on the computer screen? If you don't catch what's wrong with your pet, you'll probably be able to work it out from the medicines later.

- **Top tip:** If you really want to know what particular illness your pet has, you can always call the vet later. Best to do this in the evening when he won't be busy working and you'll get his full attention.

Paying

Most vets find it a bit embarrassing discussing the financial aspects of pet health care. Make it easy for them by not bringing any money with you, then they won't have to take any from you. A highly recommended game is to see just how much treatment you can get from a surgery without actually paying for it. If you catch them right, you can get home with a booster, wormers and a bundle of flea treatment which you can then pay for at your leisure.

- **Top tip:** Sometimes vets, no doubt under pressure from their less sympathetic bosses, can be a bit funny about the money thing. Ease their consciences by saying things like 'You surely are not going to let this animal suffer?' This usually works best if you wait until your pet is quite poorly, or hideously injured.

Repeat prescriptions

You can again save the staff at your practice from wasting time on the telephone if you don't bother to phone through orders for repeat prescriptions. It's fun to watch the nurses chuckle as they count out two or three hundred thyroid tablets in the middle of a busy surgery. You can also enjoy a bit of joking with the girls – calling out random numbers when they have got to one hundred and eighty, and that sort of thing. One thing they really love is to be asked to cut tablets into quarters for you.

- **Top tip:** If you don't like waiting in a room full of people for your prescription, pretend to run out of medication on a Saturday afternoon or a Sunday. You'll be able to have the nurse's or vet's time all to yourself.

Out-of-hours service

This is one of the most fulfilling parts of a vet's job. It's a wonderful thing that we can get twenty-four hour veterinary care for our pets for a nominal fee. In actual fact, if you have to work or play golf during the day, why not treat yourself to a personal consultation at a time to suit yourself? It may cost a little more, but think of it as business class.

Vets are dedicated professionals. Your pet's health is their main concern, and they would be disappointed in you if you didn't feel the same way. Accordingly, it doesn't matter how many weeks your dog has been coughing, or how many months your cat has had eczema, if you decide at 11 p.m. that it is causing your pet some discomfort all of a sudden, don't hesitate to phone up the duty vet. They'll be a bit bored, sitting there at the surgery all night waiting for someone to call. If you're at work anyway, you might as well see someone, don't you think?

■ **Top tip:** All vets run an emergency service. If your normal vet takes a little time to get to, why not call the closest one at night? They'll be delighted to see you.

Knowing the form

Going to the veterinary clinic is a little like going to church or having an interview at the DSS: you need to know the right responses to certain questions and situations. These are a bit of a ritual, and I doubt you would be taken seriously by many vets unless you know the right answers. Here are some examples to get you going.

When your cat gets back into its basket with alacrity at the end of a consultation:
    'You wouldn't believe the struggle we had to get her in the basket at home.'

When calling the duty vet at 3 a.m.:
    'Are you open?'

When the vet accuses your dog of being obese (choice of responses here):
    'She only gets one meal a day.'
    'It's not the food he eats.'
    'It's because she's spayed.'

When the vet asks how much exercise your hyperactive Collie gets:
    'Well, we don't actually walk him, but we've got a big garden.'

When you are about to go on holiday, your elderly dog has become ill and you don't really want to embark on treatment:
    'We don't want her to suffer.'

If your dog or cat is scratching:
    'It's not fleas.'

When your dog has an anal sac irritation:
  'It's fleas.'

When your cat has an abscess on a leg:
  'I think it's broken a leg.'

When you cat has a cat bite abscess anywhere:
  'Do you think he was bitten by a rat/squirrel/hedgehog/snake.'

When you can't think of anything else to say:
  'Do you think his nails are too long?'

When you pay the bill:
  'What did you do – gold plate him?'

Vets are generally very keen on animals, but sometimes they forget that we enjoy a little pampering as well. Perhaps someday someone will write a little guide for them along these lines, so that they can have happy clients as well as patients.

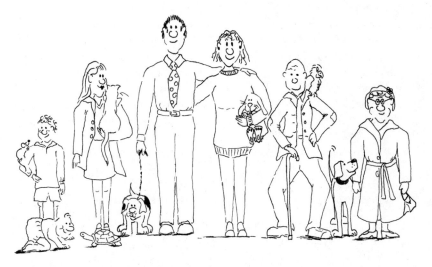

■ Don't take life too seriously

Index